Cholesterol Cures

Cholesterol Cures

More than 325 Natural Ways
to Lower Cholesterol and Live Longer
*From Almonds and Chocolate
to Garlic and Wine*

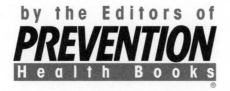

by the Editors of
PREVENTION
Health Books
®

Medical Advisor: William P. Castelli, M.D.

RODALE

Notice

This book is intended as a reference volume only, not as a medical manual. The information given here is designed to help you make informed decisions about your health. It is not intended as a substitute for any treatment that may have been prescribed by your doctor. If you suspect that you have a medical problem, we urge you to seek competent medical help.

Mention of specific companies, organizations, or authorities in this book does not imply endorsement by the publisher, nor does mention of specific companies, organizations, or authorities in the book imply that they endorse the book.

Internet addresses and telephone numbers given in this book were accurate at the time this book went to press.

Library of Congress Cataloging-in-Publication Data

Cholesterol cures : more than 325 natural ways to lower cholesterol and live longer : from almonds and chocolate to garlic and wine / by the editors of Prevention Health Books ; medical advisor, William P. Castelli.
    p.   cm.
Includes index.
ISBN 1–57954–481–9   paperback
1. Low-cholesterol diet.   2. Hypocholesteremia—Diet therapy.   I. Castelli, William P. II. Prevention Health Books.
RM237.75 .T78 2001
613.2'84—dc21   2001005500

Distributed to the book trade by St. Martin's Press

12 14 16 18 20 19 17 15 13 11   paperback

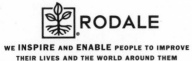

RODALE

WE INSPIRE AND ENABLE PEOPLE TO IMPROVE
THEIR LIVES AND THE WORLD AROUND THEM

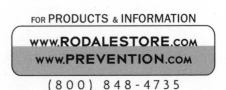

FOR PRODUCTS & INFORMATION

WWW.RODALESTORE.COM
WWW.PREVENTION.COM

(800) 848-4735

Cholesterol Cures Staff

Senior Editor: Sharon Faelten
Editors: Julia VanTine, Susan G. Berg
Writers: Richard Trubo, Lisa Delaney, Jack Forem, Jennifer Goldsmith
Interior Designers: Acey Lee, Leanne Coppola
Cover Designers: Andrew Newman, Leanne Coppola
Assistant Research Manager: Anita C. Small
Lead Researcher: Jennifer Goldsmith
Editorial Researchers: Hilton Caston, Valerie Edwards-Paulik, Theresa Fogarty, Sandra Salera Lloyd
Senior Copy Editors: Kathy D. Everleth, Amy Fisher Kovalski, Jane Sherman
Editorial Production Manager: Marilyn Hauptly
Layout Designer: Faith Hague
Product Specialist: Jodi Schaffer

Rodale Women's Health Books Group

Vice President, Editorial Director: Elizabeth Crow
Editor-in-Chief: Tammerly Booth
Writing Director: Jack Croft
Research Director: Ann Gossy Yermish
Managing Editor: Madeleine Adams
Art Director: Darlene Schneck
Office Staff: Julie Kehs Minnix, Catherine E. Strouse

CONTENTS

FOREWORD

In 1948, the town of Framingham, Massachusetts, gave the world a great gift. Half of its residents allowed doctors to study them—and, in the decades that followed, their children, grandchildren and great-grandchildren—to help the medical community unravel the mysteries of heart attack and stroke. For over 45 years, this study—known as the Framingham Heart Study—has been used to reveal the three biggest risk factors of heart disease: high levels of LDL cholesterol (the bad stuff; more about LDL in the following pages), high blood pressure and smoking. The Big Three are followed closely by overweight, lack of exercise, diabetes and stress.

Some of you might be wondering, "Aren't some people genetically predisposed to high cholesterol?" The answer is yes. But as the risk factors above show, we have to take some responsibility for having high cholesterol. After all, about 4 billion of the 5.7 billion people on the planet don't have high cholesterol. The average cholesterol level in central China, for example, is 125 milligrams/deciliter. The Masai people of Africa have cholesterol levels averaging 135 milligrams/deciliter. And in the less urban sections of Latin America, cholesterol levels hover under 150 milligrams/deciliter.

Fortunately, we can undo the harm caused by high-fat diets, inactivity and other harmful factors. That's where this book comes in. It focuses on cholesterol cures—that is, simple things virtually anyone can do to lower his or her blood cholesterol. Most of these cures focus on the foods we eat (or don't eat) and the lifestyle choices we make.

This book also provides scores of no-cholesterol and low-fat menus and recipes that can help you start *now* to lower your cholesterol—to help you reap the health benefits right away.

But be advised: There's no such thing as a magic bullet. Choosing to take antioxidant supplements, for example, or to eat more garlic while continuing to eat a high-fat diet is unlikely to affect your cholesterol for the better. And use your common sense: Consider these cures as an adjunct to a doctor's care, particularly if your cholesterol is over 200 milligrams/deciliter.

For years, the American Heart Association, the National Cholesterol Education Program of the National Heart, Lung and Blood Institute (part of the National Institutes of Health in Bethesda, Maryland) and other health organizations have run huge public service campaigns to alert the public to the risk factors that can lead to heart disease. So many of us know what we have to do to take care of our hearts. But knowledge is useless if it's not paired with action.

I encourage you to mount your own personal campaign. To do so is to validate one of the foremost conclusions of the Framingham Heart Study: that the promise—and the privilege—of good health lies in our own hands.

—William P. Castelli, M.D.
Medical director, Framingham Cardiovascular Institute
Framingham, Massachusetts

INTRODUCTION

Your Cholesterol-Reducing Action Plan

Once upon a time, when red meat, whole milk and creamery butter topped the country's culinary Hit Parade, high blood cholesterol got about as much attention from doctors and their patients as crow's-feet—it was interesting, but nothing to be alarmed about.

Not anymore. Doctors now know that high cholesterol sets the stage for a host of debilitating health conditions, including atherosclerosis (hardening of the arteries), heart attack and stroke.

To add insult to injury, high cholesterol has a nasty way of sneaking up on you (which may be why you're reading this book). If you've been ambushed by a sneak attack, you're not alone. The cholesterol levels of almost half of us exceed 200 milligrams/deciliter, even though the National Cholesterol Education Program of the National Institutes of Health has designated blood cholesterol levels of less than 200 milligrams/deciliter as desirable. About 30 percent of us are in the borderline high-risk area—technically, between 200 and 239 milligrams/deciliter. Finally, almost 20 percent of us have total cholesterol levels of 240 milligrams per deciliter or more, definitely putting us at highest risk.

But take heart. While elevated cholesterol is a significant risk factor for heart disease, it's a risk that you can control. "There are solid studies showing that watching your diet, exercising regularly and reducing your stress level can slow or even reverse atherosclerosis,"

How High Is High?

Some people can rattle off their cholesterol levels as quickly as their Social Security numbers. But if you require some translation, consult these guidelines, designated by the National Cholesterol Education Program of the National Institutes of Health and updated in 2001. (All readings are in milligrams/deciliter.)

TOTAL CHOLESTEROL

Desirable	Less than 200
Borderline high	200 to 239
High	240 or above

LDL CHOLESTEROL

Optimal	Less than 100
Near optimal/above optimal	100 to 129
Borderline high	130 to 159
High	160 to 189
Very high	190 or above

HDL CHOLESTEROL

Desirable	Above 40

says Marianne Legato, M.D., associate professor of clinical medicine at Columbia University College of Physicians and Surgeons in New York City.

If your cholesterol is within acceptable limits, this book can help you keep it there. Should it be off the charts, these doctor-recommended hints, tips and suggestions can help you knock it back, perhaps averting the need for expensive medication or even surgery.

Even if you've already been diagnosed with heart disease, there's reason for hope. Research shows that people with severe heart disease can turn their health around. One study, the Multicenter Lifestyle Demonstration Project, led by Dean Ornish, M.D., president and director of the Preventive Medicine Research Institute in Sausalito, California, was designed to determine the effectiveness and cost savings of a healthier lifestyle program. It showed that people who were eligible for bypass surgery or angioplasty were able to avoid it for at least three years by making lifestyle changes recommended in hospital programs that followed Dr. Ornish's guidelines.

A previous study, the Lifestyle Heart Trial, also led by Dr. Ornish, concluded that people with heart disease can often stop or even reverse their conditions with lifestyle changes alone. Most likely, you can do it, too.

Why You Should Wage a Plaque Attack

To fire up your resolve, here's a list of the most significant benefits of reducing your cholesterol.

You can slow or even reverse the progression of atherosclerosis. In atherosclerosis, fatty deposits called plaques stick to the walls of the coronary arteries, the vessels that supply oxygen-rich blood to the heart. Atherosclerosis can lead to coronary heart disease, or blockages in the coronary arteries. If left untreated, these blockages can choke off the heart's supply of blood, leading to chest pain (angina), heart attack, or even death.

Lowering your cholesterol can reduce your chances of atherosclerosis and coronary heart disease. One landmark study, the Lipid Research Clinics Coronary Primary Prevention Trial, found that for each 1 percent you lower your total cholesterol, the probability of developing coronary heart disease or having a heart attack falls by 2 percent. The same study found that as cholesterol levels dip, so does the incidence of angina and the need for coronary bypass surgery.

You can reduce or eliminate your reliance on cholesterol-lowering medication. While people with extremely high cholesterol may need cholesterol-lowering drugs—most notably statin drugs like lovastatin (Mevacor) and simvastatin (Zocor)—"drugs are the second line of defense," says John McDougall, M.D., creator and head of the McDougall Program at St. Helena Hospital in Santa Rosa, California. "Diet and lifestyle changes are the foundation for recovering from coronary heart disease."

You can reduce your risk of stroke. One study found that elevated cholesterol can produce abnormal amounts of a chemical that can cause spasms in the carotid artery in the neck, which supplies blood to the brain. If these spasms interrupt blood flow, they could cause a mini-stroke, or transient ischemic attack. Additionally, if

UPDATED GOVERNMENT CHOLESTEROL GUIDELINES CALL FOR MORE ATTENTION TO DIET AND LIFESTYLE

Lifestyle changes—the clinician's shorthand for healthy eating, regular exercise and weight control—are the first line of defense against high cholesterol and heart disease.

That's the word from the National Cholesterol Education Program's Adult Treatment Panel III (ATP III) report, issued May 14, 2001, which contains revised guidelines for preventing and treating high cholesterol. The National Cholesterol Education Program is an initiative of the National Heart, Lung, and Blood Institute, part of the National Institutes of Health.

The ATP III guidelines also recommend:

- Treating high cholesterol more aggressively in people with type 2 diabetes. They're at particularly high risk of dying from a heart attack.
- Setting a new level at which low HDL cholesterol becomes a risk factor for heart disease. Reflecting recent findings about the strong link between low HDL and heart disease, low HDL is now defined as being below 40 milligrams/deciliter, up from 35 milligrams/deciliter.
- Advocating a more in-depth initial test for high cholesterol. The first test should be a complete lipoprotein profile—including total, HDL and LDL cholesterol and triglyceride levels—rather than just total and HDL cholesterol.

The NIH has developed an online calculator to help men and women determine their risk for heart attack over the next ten years. To find it, go

deposits of excess LDL in an artery break free, they can cause a blood clot that blocks blood flow to the brain, triggering a stroke.

If you have diabetes, you can troubleshoot potential problems. Some research suggests that both women and men with diabetes have about twice the coronary heart disease risk of the general population. People with diabetes who have had a coronary event are also twice as likely to suffer repeat problems, such as heart attacks, angina and the need for bypass surgery. People with diabetes also tend to have high levels of triglycerides, another blood fat implicated in coronary heart disease. If you have diabetes, lowering your choto their Web site at http://rover.nhlbi.nih.gov/guidelines/cholesterol/ and click on "patients."

Lifestyle changes alone can lower cholesterol levels in some folks with elevated cholesterol. But more beans, greens and brisk walks can also benefit the 13 million men and women who take cholesterol-lowering drugs, according to the authors of the report.

Compared with the previous ATP report, issued in 1993, ATP III places more emphasis on "therapeutic lifestyle changes," or TLC—rather than medication—as the first treatment for elevated cholesterol and particularly for "bad" LDL cholesterol, which is a major cause of coronary heart disease.

There are four components of TLC.

- To reduce intake of saturated fat—the artery-clogging fat found in foods like bacon, butter and full-fat cheese—to less than 7 percent of total daily calories and to limit intake of dietary cholesterol to no more than 200 milligrams a day.
- To get 10 to 25 grams (2 to 5 teaspoons) per day of soluble fiber, found in foods such as cereal grains, beans, fruits and vegetables. It also encourages the use of foods that contain sterols and stanols. These plant substances are found in some types of spreads and salad dressings, such as Benecol and Take Control.
- To get at least 30 minutes of physical activity a day.
- To lose weight.

The information and advice given in this book has been updated and revised to help you achieve all of those heart-healthy diet and lifestyle goals.

lesterol and controlling other risk factors such as high blood pressure and overweight can cut the chances of developing diabetes-related heart and blood vessel problems.

You can increase your quantity of life. The renowned Framingham Heart Study, which has tracked the health of the residents of Framingham, Massachusetts, for more than four decades, has shown that the lower cholesterol levels fall, the lower the chance of heart attack and sudden death.

You can enhance your quality of life. Taking charge of elevated cholesterol now could mean the difference between a future of shuttling to and from the doctor's office (or the hospital) and enjoying a full, happy, healthy life.

A Cholesterol Primer

Cholesterol is a soft, waxy substance found in every human cell, in blood and in food. The kind found in food is called dietary cholesterol. Only animal-based foods such as meat and dairy products contain dietary cholesterol; it's not found in plant-based foods such as fruits, vegetables, beans and grains.

Believe it or not, cholesterol isn't as evil as you might think. Your body actually needs the stuff, and your cells make what they need. Your liver, for example, uses cholesterol to make bile acids, which help you digest food.

But too much cholesterol circulating in your blood can lead to trouble. One study, the Multiple Risk Factor Intervention Trial, evaluated nearly 360,000 American men, none of whom had yet experi-

---

MEN: LOWER YOUR CHOLESTEROL, IMPROVE YOUR LOVE LIFE?

Men with high total cholesterol and low levels of good HDL cholesterol may be prime candidates for erectile difficulty, several studies show.

In one study, researchers gave a group of 3,371 men physical exams, including cholesterol tests. Each man visited the clinic twice, with an average of 22 months between visits.

In that time, 71 men developed difficulty achieving or maintaining erections. Men with total cholesterol levels above 240 milligrams/deciliter were 83 percent more likely to experience the problem than men whose total cholesterol was below 180 milligrams/deciliter. Also, men whose HDL exceeded 60 milligrams/deciliter were 70 percent less likely to have difficulty than men whose HDL was below 30 milligrams/deciliter. Atherosclerosis may cause the problem by reducing blood flow to the penis, the researchers speculated.

Another study, which examined the various causes of erectile difficulty in Massachusetts men, found that the men's risk rose as their HDL levels dipped.

WILL HRT HELP? IT DEPENDS

Before they reach menopause, women have significantly lower rates of coronary heart disease than men of the same ages. Why? In a word: estrogen. This female sex hormone appears to raise women's stores of heart-healthy HDL cholesterol. "Women tend to have higher HDL than men, which may be why they have less heart disease than men—at least in their premenopausal years," says Peter Wood, D.Sc., Ph.D., professor emeritus of medicine at Stanford University School of Medicine.

After the onset of menopause, a woman's levels of total and LDL cholesterol rise and her HDL wanes, most likely due to a dwindling supply of estrogen. "Postmenopausal women's heart attack rates eventually catch up with those of men their ages," says William P. Castelli, M.D., medical director of the Framingham Cardiovascular Institute, a wellness program at Metro West Medical Center in Massachusetts. But take heart: "Women can raise their HDL by quitting smoking, losing weight and getting regular exercise," he says.

For many women and their doctors, hormone replacement therapy (HRT, comprised of estrogen or estrogen and progesterone) is the treatment of choice for the changes typically associated with menopause, from temporary discomforts like hot flashes to long-term consequences like decreasing bone density. HRT was once considered beneficial to women's heart health, but new evidence suggests that for some women, the reverse may be true. One large study suggested that it seems to increase the risk of death in women who already have heart disease when they begin treatment. A more definitive verdict on HRT won't be in until 2005, when larger studies of estrogen and heart health are completed. But for now, many doctors think that HRT is both safe and beneficial if a woman has risk factors for heart disease but hasn't developed the condition yet.

Your best bet? "Discuss HRT with your doctor before menopause so that you'll have a plan in place once it happens," advises Debra Judelson, M.D., medical director of the Women's Heart Institute at the Cardiovascular Medical Group in Los Angeles.

---

enced a heart attack. After seven years, the investigators found that the risk of dying of coronary heart disease was two times higher in men with total cholesterol above 220 milligrams/deciliter than in men with total cholesterol of 180 milligrams/deciliter or less. Men with readings of 245 milligrams/deciliter had triple the risk.

Studies of women show that before menopause, their levels of blood cholesterol tend to average about ten points lower than men's. At menopause, however, the gap closes, and women seem to run the same risk as men.

More Than One Kind of Blood Fat Is Involved

Cholesterol doesn't dissolve in blood, so it can't get to where the body needs it on its own. It has to hitch a ride on special carriers called lipoproteins. There are two major types: low-density lipoprotein (LDL) and high-density lipoprotein (HDL). LDL, the "bad" type, is packed with cholesterol, while HDL, the "good" cholesterol, is mostly protein.

If there's too much LDL in your blood, it gets deposited on the walls of your arteries as fatty clumps. If these clumps break free, they can cause the blood to clot. A clot that cuts off the flow of blood to the heart can cause a heart attack; a clot that blocks blood flow to the brain can trigger a stroke.

HDL, on the other hand, is a cardiovascular hero. It patrols your arteries, hauling cholesterol away from them and carrying it to the liver for dumping. Experts agree that the higher your level of HDL, the better your cardiovascular health is likely to be. One study has concluded that for each one milligram/deciliter rise in HDL, the risk of coronary heart disease declines by 2 to 3 percent.

Cardiology researchers in Connecticut think that low levels of HDL may indicate future heart trouble just as strongly as high LDL levels do, so doctors and their patients need to focus more on increasing HDL levels. Most people and their doctors are aware of the role of eating healthier and exercising more, and the introduction of the statin drugs in the past decade has helped. But now doctors feel that even more can be done.

"People are asking, What more can we do?" says Daniel J. Diver, M.D., head of cardiology at Saint Francis Hospital and Medical Center in Hartford, Connecticut. The answer is to increase HDL levels. Research has shown that HDL levels are the best gauge of long-term survival in people who have undergone bypass surgery. "In the past few years," Dr. Diver says, "HDL has emerged as an independent predictor of heart disease."

Whenever you have a cholesterol test, the lab will also measure triclygerides, since many people with high triglycerides have high LDL or low HDL levels. Triglyceride levels of less than 150 milligrams per deciliter are considered desirable.

Additionally, it's a good idea to know your level of lipoprotein(a), or LP(a). LP(a) is a chunk of cholesterol coated with protein, and it's found only in the blood of hedgehogs, certain monkeys—and people. Researchers at Oxford University in England found that among people who had heart disease or who had survived a heart attack, those who had the highest levels of LP(a) also had a 70 percent greater risk of having a heart attack over a ten-year period than those with the lowest levels. Levels starting at 30 milligrams/deciliter seem to raise risks. The Framingham Heart Study found that having levels of about 30 milligrams/deciliter doubled the risk of heart attack in 3,000 women, so LP(a) tests are something to consider if you're female or have heart disease or a family history of premature coronary artery disease or stroke.

What's Your Ratio?

Most likely, you're familiar with your total cholesterol, or the sum of your HDL and LDL values and those of other blood fats. To see if your blood fats fall within a desirable range, your doctor will determine your cholesterol ratio—that is, your total cholesterol divided by your HDL number. The theory is that combining the levels into one number will give you an overall look at your individual heart disease risk. Experts agree that the ideal ratio is 3.5 to 1 or lower, although many feel that it's even more important to pay attention to the individual values, since levels of both LDL and HDL play a role in predicting heart health.

Let's say you learn that your total cholesterol is 250 milligrams/deciliter and your HDL is 50 milligrams/deciliter (above the new desired minimum of 40 milligrams/deciliter). Dividing your total cholesterol (250) by your HDL (50) gives you a ratio of 5 to 1. But cutting your total cholesterol to 200 milligrams/deciliter (the new desired maximum) while holding your HDL at 50 milligrams/deciliter will shrink your ratio to a more desirable 4 to 1. In fact, doctors participating in the Physicians' Health Study—an ongoing study of more than 22,000 American doctors conducted at Harvard Medical School and Brigham and Women's Hospital in Boston—found that cutting just one unit from their ratios of total to HDL cholesterol slashed their heart attack risk by 53 percent!

A Cornucopia of Natural Cholesterol "Prescriptions"

If your cholesterol is high, one recourse is to take cholesterol-lowering drugs, which can do a great deal to keep LDL levels in check. Unfortunately, they come at a price. Since they're metabolized

---

FIVE PROVEN WAYS TO LOWER YOUR CHOLESTEROL

There are dozens of options, major and minor, for lowering your cholesterol. To help you focus and prioritize your choices, try this simple five-step approach.

1. Choose your fats wisely. Most people now get about 37 percent of total calories from fat, down from 42 percent in the 1960s. This is great news, since consuming too much fat, particularly saturated fat, has been linked to an increased risk of coronary heart disease. But we still have a way to go: The American Heart Association recommends getting no more than 30 percent of calories from fat. Other experts suggest 25 percent or even less.

While cutting back on saturated fat is an excellent move, it's actually a better idea to eat more monounsaturated fat—found in olive and canola oils, most nuts (almonds, walnuts, peanuts and peanut butter, and pecans), and avocados—than to eliminate all fat. In one study, a diet high in monounsaturated fat lowered triglycerides in overweight men.

2. Get serious about losing weight. People who follow low-fat, low-cholesterol diets and lose excess weight tend to have an easier time reducing their levels of total and LDL cholesterol than people who don't drop the extra pounds, says Margo Denke, M.D., associate professor of medicine in the Center for Human Nutrition at the University of Texas Southwestern Medical Center in Dallas. Being overweight seems to disrupt the normal metabolism of fats, which means that even if you eat less fat (a common first step in trying to clobber cholesterol), you won't get the biggest heart benefits unless you lose weight.

One study of 150 overweight people concluded that those who lose just 10 to 15 percent of excess body weight—and keep it off—may afford themselves long-term protection from coronary heart disease.

in the liver, you have to be monitored regularly for liver damage. So anything that can be done to lower cholesterol naturally can help minimize your doctor's need to prescribe a drug.

In the chapters that follow, you'll read about practical, expert-recommended strategies that can help you wallop high cholesterol without the use of prescription drugs. Some of these tactics may sound familiar; others are on the cutting edge of medical research. Provided that your physician gives you the green light, you can add

---

Dropping extra pounds may also boost HDL cholesterol. In a study of 2,400 people, women experienced a 2 percent increase in LDL and a 2 percent drop in HDL for every five pounds they gained. "Being overweight is the most common cause of low HDL in women," says Dr. Denke. "It's important to get down to an ideal body weight to bring HDL back up."

Research from the landmark Framingham Heart Study shows that weight loss helps your health in other ways. Taking off 1 to 2 pounds a year—and maintaining the loss—may cut your risk of high blood pressure by 25 percent and of diabetes by 35 percent.

3. Step up your efforts to exercise. Researchers at Stanford University found that people who teamed exercise with a low-fat diet doubled their LDL reduction. They participated in 30 minutes of moderate exercise at least three times a week. Accumulating 45 to 60 minutes of moderate-intensity activity at least five days a week also helps you lose weight.

4. If you smoke, quit once and for all. Smoking can lead to atherosclerosis and can reduce HDL by as much as 15 percent. Within two years after you quit, however, your risk of heart disease is about the same as that of someone who never smoked, says Lori Mosca, M.D., Ph.D., director of preventive cardiology research and education at the University of Michigan in Ann Arbor. So quitting can significantly improve your cholesterol profile.

"Quitting smoking can reverse the negative effect on HDL in just 60 days," explains Robert Rosenson, M.D., director of the Preventive Cardiology Center at Rush–Presbyterian–St. Luke's Medical Center in Chicago.

5. Reduce your stress levels. Chronic stress may raise levels of homocysteine, an amino acid that's been linked to increased heart disease risk in men and women. So, keeping cool may help keep the lid on your cholesterol.

virtually all of these strategies to your daily routine with a minimum of time, money and effort.

Along the way, you'll gain a wealth of practical information that can help you achieve your ultimate goal—a heart-healthy cholesterol level. You'll discover:

- How olives, peanut butter, avocados and other indulgences can help boost your good cholesterol and lower your bad cholesterol
- Why folks in certain parts of the world seem to enjoy better heart health than we do, and why some experts continue to steer us toward the kinds of foods favored in Mediterranean diets
- Ongoing research that suggests certain vitamins and minerals may help reduce cholesterol and protect against coronary heart disease
- Tips from chefs who've mastered the art of reducing fat and cholesterol in their recipes without reducing flavor
- A comprehensive table of the total and saturated fat contents of 500 common foods

As a bonus, we've devised a time-tested, cholesterol-busting menu plan designed to drop your total cholesterol 30 points in 30 days while improving your HDL reading. You'll find this plan—created by a Rodale nutritionist, approved by a top registered dietitian, and tested by a veteran health book editor—as delicious as it is effective.

Think of this plan as your own personal cholesterol-reduction tool. The sooner you put it to work, the sooner you'll reap your reward: a strong, healthy heart primed to provide years of vibrant living.

ALCOHOL

It's an Option, Not a "Must"

Drinking protects your heart, right?

Wrong. Or at least not quite right.

But that's the message some Americans came away with some years ago, when a few studies indicated that moderate drinking is associated with reduced risk of coronary heart disease. The truth is, deciding whether to imbibe to protect your heart isn't as simple as deciding to eat less saturated fat and more soluble fiber.

On the one hand, there's evidence that moderate consumption of alcohol can help reduce the risk of coronary heart disease as well as help raise levels of "good" HDL cholesterol. On the other hand, many experts question the wisdom of encouraging people to drink for their health. In fact, some health professionals suggest that the decision to drink moderately to benefit heart health be made with the guidance of a physician. Experts are equally clear on another point: If you don't drink, don't start. This chapter can help you make an informed decision about the benefits—and risks—of moderate drinking to raise HDL and lower heart disease risk.

The Benefits of Limited Consumption

Two studies, in particular, looked at the relationship between drinking habits and cholesterol and triglyceride levels in women. One study, conducted in Finland, reviewed the drinking habits of 274 healthy, middle-aged women with different drinking habits and then did a follow-up analysis of nonalcoholic drinking women. Among the women studied, total and HDL cholesterol levels improved, but LDL levels did not. The effect was most noticeable in women who reported drinking between $\frac{2}{3}$ ounce and almost $1\frac{1}{2}$ ounces of alcohol a day—about the equivalent of a small glass of wine, half a can of beer, or a mixed drink. When they drank more than $1\frac{1}{2}$ ounces, all cholesterol values increased except for LDL. When the women then abstained for two weeks, their HDL dropped and their LDL cholesterol increased.

Other researchers studied the effect of slightly higher alcohol consumption on cardiovascular risk factors in women so they could compare the effect to that previously observed in men. In this study, the women—who were either postmenopausal or premenopausal and taking oral contraceptives—drank three glasses a day of either red wine or grape juice with dinner for three weeks. After three weeks, the researchers took blood samples 1 hour before dinner and then at 2- or 4-hour intervals for up to 19 hours after dinner. In both premenopausal and postmenopausal women, levels of both triglycerides and very low density lipoprotein (VLDL, an even more harmful type of LDL) peaked 3 hours after a dinner with wine. In addition, after drinking wine, the premenopausal women had a 12 percent increase in overall HDL cholesterol levels, and the postmenopausal women's LDL cholesterol levels decreased by the same amount, when compared with grape juice consumption. The response of postmenopausal women to alcohol resembled the response found in earlier studies in men.

Why does moderate alcohol consumption seem to beneficially raise HDL cholesterol? Experts aren't sure. "We don't entirely understand the effect of alcohol on HDL," says Peter O. Kwiterovich Jr., M.D., professor of medicine and director of the Lipid Research and Atherosclerosis Unit at Johns Hopkins University School of Medicine in Baltimore. "But it's pretty clear from epidemiological studies that people who drink moderately do better than people who don't drink at all."

"The data are clear that a drink or two a day lowers your heart attack risk," agrees William P. Castelli, M.D., medical director of the

Framingham Cardiovascular Institute, a wellness program at Metro West Medical Center in Massachusetts.

According to data from the second National Health and Nutrition Examination Survey, average levels of HDL cholesterol were higher among drinkers than among abstainers, no matter what their age, sex or race. Also, as alcohol consumption increased, so did HDL levels—an average increase of 5.1 milligrams/deciliter for daily or weekly use. (This study suggests reducing your risk of coronary heart disease by means other than alcohol consumption, however.)

For seven years, the Multiple Risk Factor Intervention Trial followed a subgroup consisting of 11,688 middle-aged men who were at high risk for heart disease. During that time, those who consumed about two drinks per day (with each drink equal to 4 ounces of wine, 12 ounces of beer or 1.5 ounces of 80-proof spirits) had higher HDL levels than nondrinkers. This alcohol intake seemed largely responsible for a 22 percent reduced chance of death from heart disease, researchers said.

Researchers at Kaiser Permanente Medical Center in Oakland, California, studied the alcohol consumption patterns of nearly 129,000 people. Those who had one to two drinks a day were 30 percent less likely to die from coronary heart disease than those who did not drink. But people who had six or more drinks a day had a 60 percent greater risk of death from noncardiovascular causes than nondrinkers.

Dr. Kwiterovich and his colleagues had 56 men with low levels of HDL either drink one beer a day or abstain from alcohol. After two months, there were no differences in HDL levels between the two groups. But the beer drinkers experienced a 10 percent increase in apolipoprotein A-1, the major protein component of HDL. This protein is believed to help extract cholesterol from the cells and move it to the liver for excretion. Alcohol also makes blood platelets less sticky, which cuts the risk of clot formation and reduces the risk of heart attack, and raises blood levels of an enzyme called tissue-type plasminogen activator, or tPA, which helps keep blood clots from forming.

Researchers at Harvard University and Brigham and Women's Hospital in Boston measured blood levels of tPA in 631 male doctors. These doctors—participants in the Physicians' Health Study, a study of 22,000 American doctors—gave blood samples and reported on their drinking habits. Researchers found that tPA levels rose with drinking frequency. The doctors who consumed two or more drinks a day had 35 percent higher levels of tPA than doctors who rarely or never drank. What's more, the doctors who drank more had significantly higher levels of HDL cholesterol than the doctors who didn't.

Not a Magic Bullet

If you think that simply hoisting a beer stein or sipping your favorite Bordeaux will have a beneficial effect on your cholesterol level, think again. "Two glasses of wine a day will have a modest effect on your HDL, and even that modest effect is beneficial," says Dr. Castelli. "But if you're looking for a magic bullet, this isn't it."

Further, overimbibing to benefit your cholesterol level is risky, say experts. "Alcohol is like coffee—it has some theoretical benefits and some potential risks," says Neal Barnard, M.D., president of the Physicians Committee for Responsible Medicine in Washington, D.C. Risks include developing certain cancers and provoking cardiac arrhythmias, cirrhosis of the liver and high blood pressure, says Dr. Castelli.

"It appears that women have an increased risk of breast cancer from increased alcohol consumption, even at the moderate levels recommended as potentially beneficial for heart disease," says Marla Mendelson, M.D., assistant professor of medicine at Northwestern University Medical School in Chicago. "So women who have a significant risk of developing breast cancer have to think twice about drinking."

There are other issues to consider. "If you have high blood pressure, alcohol can raise it more," says Frederic J. Pashkow, M.D., cardiologist at the Cleveland Clinic Foundation in Ohio and author of *50 Essential Things to Do When the Doctor Says It's Heart Disease*.

What's more, alcohol can actually raise triglycerides by lowering the concentration of an enzyme used to break them down. "Even having a glass of wine with dinner every night can substantially raise triglycerides in people who are overweight or who have hereditary triglyceride problems," says Thomas Bersot, M.D., associate professor of medicine at the University of California, San Francisco.

The bottom line? If you choose to imbibe, do so in moderation—and if you don't drink, don't start, says Margo Denke, M.D., associate professor of medicine in the Center for Human Nutrition at the University of Texas Southwestern Medical Center at Dallas.

Dr. Barnard agrees. "I suggest that people follow a low-fat diet. I'm not sure that adding alcohol to that would be helpful."

See also Grape Juice, Wine

~❦~
_____

ALMONDS

A Handful of Health

In ancient Greece, the almond was so popular that it was nicknamed the Greek nut. And centuries later, we still crave this sweet, crunchy nut, whether as a snack or as an ingredient in many main dishes and desserts.

But almonds are more than just delicious. These nuts are loaded with calcium, which keeps bones and teeth strong; vitamin E, an antioxidant vitamin thought to reduce the risk of heart disease and certain types of cancer; and magnesium, which helps regulate blood pressure.

Almonds, and nuts in general, are also high in monounsaturated fat, which has been shown to lower total and "bad" LDL cholesterol without detrimentally affecting the "good" HDL cholesterol. Nearly two-thirds (65 percent) of the total fat of almonds is monounsaturated.

The Heart-Healthy Fat

Researchers at Loma Linda University in California examined the link between eating nuts—including almonds, walnuts and peanuts—and a reduced risk of heart disease in more than 31,000 Seventh-Day Adventists. The researchers found that those who ate nuts more than four times a week had about half the risk of suffering a heart attack (fatal or nonfatal) of those who ate nuts less than once a week. Twenty-nine percent of the nuts consumed were almonds.

"There are several possible reasons why almonds and other nuts seem to be capable of lowering blood cholesterol levels," says Gary E. Fraser, M.D., Ph.D., professor of medicine at Loma Linda University School of Public Health and head of the study. "Almost certainly, nuts' high level of monounsaturated fat is a major factor. But nuts are also a very good source of an amino acid called arginine, which is a dietary precursor of a chemical called nitric oxide, a major EDRF (en-

Heart-Healthy ♡
Indulgences

MIXED NUTS: MULTIPLE BENEFITS

Almonds aren't the only nuts that have proven health benefits. Walnuts have similar properties, and even macadamia nuts—the "caviar" of nutty snacks—can be beneficial, if you don't go nuts. (We had to say it.)

Research has consistently shown that people who eat a lot of nuts have a much lower risk of heart disease. Consider results from the landmark Nurses' Health Study, for example: The heart attack risk of women who ate the most nuts (about 5 ounces a week) was half that of those who rarely ate them.

Researchers aren't quite sure what makes nuts so heart-friendly. It's thought that the unsaturated fats, magnesium, copper, folate, protein, potassium, fiber and vitamin E may all be part of the protective package.

Still, at about 180 calories per ounce, nuts are a high-calorie treat. To be good to your heart and your waistline, eat small amounts (about an ounce) two to five times a week.

Nuts aren't just for eating out of a bowl or bag, though. Here are some other ways to enjoy them.

- For the ultimate dessert, try two or three chocolate-covered macadamia nuts.
- Roast nuts lightly in your toaster oven to bring out the flavor.
- Toss about ½ cup of nuts into homemade bread.
- Add them to salads and cooked vegetables.
- For a snack, combine almonds and dried dates.
- Add nuts to hot or cold cereal, yogurt and even pasta dishes.

dothelium-derived relaxing factor)." This chemical, which is released in the lining of the artery wall, seems to help prevent atherosclerosis, explains Dr. Fraser.

One of the most comprehensive studies of the almond/cholesterol link was conducted by Gene A. Spiller, D.Sc., Ph.D., director of the Health Research and Studies Center in Los Altos, California, and author of *The Superpyramid Eating Program.* In Dr. Spiller's study, 26 men and women ate a low-fat, low-cholesterol diet brimming with vegetables, fruits, grains, beans and low-fat dairy products for nine weeks. They avoided foods such as butter, margarine, fatty fish, most meats and ice cream. After following this low-fat baseline diet for two weeks, the participants also began eating about three ounces of raw almonds a day and using almond oil instead of other vegetable oils.

When the participants added almonds to their diet, their total daily fat intake rose from 67 to 90 grams a day; about 37 percent of their daily calories came from fat. But after three weeks of following the almond-rich diet, these folks' average total cholesterol plummeted from 235 to 215 milligrams/deciliter. What's more, their average LDL cholesterol fell 21 points—from 154 to 133 milligrams/deciliter. Their HDL cholesterol levels remained steady.

Why did the total and LDL cholesterol levels of these men and women decline, despite their eating more fat? Perhaps because the extra fat derived from the almonds is monounsaturated, speculate Dr. Spiller and his colleagues. "But if these men and women had been getting 40 percent of their calories from mostly saturated fat—if they had had bacon for breakfast, steak for dinner and butter on their bread—you wouldn't want to add many almonds on top of that," says Dr. Spiller. Dr. Spiller's study further concluded that following a diet higher in total fat than usually recommended can still help lower cholesterol if the diet is high in plant foods.

Nutty Ways to Enjoy Almonds

Grabbing a fistful of raw, unsalted almonds is one way to take advantage of these nuts' power to lower cholesterol. Here are some others.

• To enjoy the flavor of almonds without the added fat or salt of the canned kind, toast the nuts yourself. Here's how: Spread whole raw almonds in a single layer across a shallow pan. Place the pan in a cold oven, then heat to 350°. Stir the nuts occasionally. When they're lightly toasted (8 to 12 minutes), remove from the pan and cool.

You can microwave almonds, too. Place ½ cup of raw almonds on a microwave-safe plate or bowl. Then zap the almonds for two to six minutes on high power, stirring once a minute. Let cool.

• Sprinkle your cereal, waffles or pancakes with slivered almonds. Or stir ground-up almonds into fat-free or low-fat yogurt.

• "Sprinkle almonds in your salads," says Dr. Spiller. To prepare almonds for salads, toss raw almonds into a pot of boiling water for about a minute (a cooking method called blanching). Drain the almonds and remove the skin, suggests Dr. Spiller. Then toast the nuts as above, chop and add to the greens.

• Add almonds to a variety of soups, including vegetable soup, suggests Dr. Spiller. "Grind or chop the almonds before adding to the soup," he advises.

• Stir chopped or ground-up almonds into cooked vegetables and pasta dishes.

• Replace small amounts of meat, fish or chicken in main dish casseroles with ground almonds. You'll boost your consumption of healthier monounsaturated fat while you reduce your intake of saturated fat.

Go Nuts without Gaining Weight

One ounce of almonds (about 20 to 25 nuts) contains about 170 calories. So these nuts aren't exactly a low-calorie snack. But you don't have to deprive yourself of almonds' cholesterol-busting potential, says Dr. Spiller. Just indulge wisely.

"Some people are afraid they'll gain weight if they add almonds to their diets," says Dr. Spiller. "But their weight often stays the same, probably because as they eat more almonds, they tend to cut down on other foods and replace animal protein with plant protein. You should do the same."

If you're over your desirable weight, however, don't go nuts over almonds, advises Dr. Spiller. "Don't follow your big meal of the day with three ounces of almonds," he says. "Add almonds to your diet in place of something else."

∾✲৶

ANTIOXIDANTS

The Plaque-Attacking Cardio-Nutrients

Low in fat, high in fiber and cholesterol-free, fruits and veggies are crucial components of a heart-healthy diet. But there may be another reason to load up on produce. There's evidence that the antioxidant nutrients—vitamins C and E and beta-carotene, which converts to vitamin A in the body—may protect against high blood cholesterol levels. These "supernutrients," which are abundant in fresh fruits and vegetables, may even help prevent heart disease.

Indeed, an Australian study showed the promising effects of vitamin C on cholesterol levels. Researchers looked at the effect of taking 2,000 milligrams of vitamin C daily on various indicators of heart health, including cholesterol, in 18 healthy men whose vitamin C levels were low but still normal. Total cholesterol levels were 10 percent lower in men who received the vitamin C compared with those of men who got a placebo (an inactive, look-alike pill), although total cholesterol/HDL ratios were not significantly different.

There's more evidence. In a large British study, researchers looked at the combined effects of cholesterol-lowering therapy and antioxidant vitamin supplements. They focused on men and women ages 40 to 80 who were considered to be at high risk of dying from heart disease. Some received simvastatin (Zocor), a cholesterol-lowering drug (40 milligrams a day); others received a placebo plus antioxidant vitamins (600 milligrams of vitamin E, 250 milligrams of vitamin C, and 20 milligrams of beta-carotene daily) or a placebo alone. All were checked at various intervals for at least five years.

After 30 months, both total cholesterol and LDL cholesterol levels fell in the first two groups. Researchers say that among the type of people included in the study, the incidence rate of fatal heart attacks dropped by 2.4 percent a year. They concluded that people at highest risk for heart disease benefit from both cholesterol-lowering therapy and antioxidant vitamin supplements.

Those are just two of the numerous studies that associate a high intake of antioxidant vitamins with a lower risk of coronary heart disease and improvement in cholesterol. Many of those studies have found that these benefits occur with doses that are higher than the Daily Values (DVs) for the nutrients. The DV for vitamin C is 60 milligrams; for vitamin E, it's 30 international units. While there is no DV for beta-carotene, some experts recommend consuming just 5 to 6 milligrams daily from foods.

Some authorities recommend taking supplements of vitamins C and E to bridge the gap between the DVs and these theoretically therapeutic doses, but supplementation with beta-carotene is not generally recommended. Others consider supplements a "promising but unproven" means of lowering the risk of cardiovascular disease.

Experts say, however, that gulping down antioxidant supplements won't compensate for a high-fat, artery-clogging diet. The best way to lower your cholesterol—and protect your heart—is to follow a low-fat, low-cholesterol diet, they say. Here's how antioxidants may help.

The Antioxidant-Cholesterol Link

Experts believe that antioxidants help thwart a number of chronic illnesses, including heart disease, by foiling the activity of free radicals. Damage from these cell-damaging chemical compounds, which are produced both inside and outside the body, can eventually lead to disease, including heart disease. Antioxidant vitamins may help stem this cellular damage.

Furthermore, antioxidants may help boost "good" HDL cholesterol and help artery-clogging LDL cholesterol resist oxidation, a chemical process that researchers believe increases the likelihood that LDL will collect in the arteries.

"LDL is the major cholesterol-carrying molecule in the bloodstream," says Thomas Bersot, M.D., associate professor of medicine at the University of California, San Francisco. Oxidized LDL is more likely to be trapped by macrophages, a type of cell in the walls of the arteries. When LDL starts to collect inside the macrophages, it sets up a chemical chain reaction that can accelerate oxidation and other artery-clogging processes.

"The accumulation of LDL in the macrophages initiates the entire

---

GOOD FOOD SOURCES OF ANTIOXIDANTS

What do clams, kale and cantaloupe have in common? They're all brimming with antioxidant vitamins. Here's a short list of antioxidant-rich fare.

VITAMIN C

Broccoli	Mangoes
Brussels sprouts	Oranges
Cantaloupe	Papaya
Cauliflower	Peppers
Clams	Potatoes
Grapefruit	Watermelon
Green peppers	

VITAMIN E

Asparagus	Sunflower seeds
Cereal (fortified)	Sweet potatoes
Kale	Vegetable oil
Liver	Wheat germ
Nuts	Whole grain products
Pumpkin seeds	

BETA-CAROTENE

Apricots	Peaches
Cantaloupe	Spinach
Carrots	Sweet potatoes
Mangoes	Tomatoes
Papaya	Yellow squash

---

cascade of events in atherosclerosis," says Dr. Bersot. "If you can prevent LDL from oxidizing, you may reduce the risk of developing hardening of the arteries."

Antioxidants to the Rescue

A number of studies have demonstrated an association between a higher intake of antioxidant supplements—particularly vitamins C and E—and a lower risk of heart disease.

Researchers in the Health Professionals Study, conducted at Harvard

Heart-Healthy♡
Indulgences

GUACAMOLE: THE GREAT GREEN FAT FIGHTER

Next time you dine at a Mexican restaurant, pass up the sour cream in favor of the guacamole. Avocado, the main ingredient in guacamole, is a very rich source of the antioxidant glutathione. Tests conducted at Louisiana State University showed that glutathione can help to block the absorption of harmful fat in the intestinal tract. It also protects the DNA in cells from free radical damage, which has been linked to aging. Avocados contain at least three times more glutathione than any other fruit.

Avocados are also high in unsaturated fat, and the U.S. government's new dietary guidelines suggest that a diet based on moderate amounts of foods high in unsaturated fats can also help keep cholesterol low and offer some protection against heart disease.

Don't kid yourself, though: Eating too much fat of any kind means eating more calories than you need. Also, avocado can't completely combat the effects of the saturated fat from the refried beans and deep-fried chips in your Mexican meal.

To benefit your waistline and your heart, use the following strategies.

• When you make guacamole at home, cut the fat by using tomatillos (Mexican green tomatoes) in place of some of the avocados.
• Eat less of other fatty foods while you're enjoying your guacamole.

Medical School and the Harvard School of Public Health, followed 40,000 healthy male health care workers for four years, tracking how many developed heart disease during that time. They found that the men who consumed the most vitamin E had a lower risk of heart disease. Men who took 100 or more international units of vitamin E for at least two years cut their risk of heart disease by 37 percent compared with men who did not take any supplements.

A parallel Harvard study evaluated more than 87,000 healthy female nurses for eight years. Women who consumed the most vitamin E were found to have a 34 percent reduced risk of developing heart disease compared with women who consumed the least vitamin E.

Women who had taken vitamin E supplements for at least two years had a 41 percent lower chance of developing coronary disease than those who hadn't taken supplements. And women who consumed the most beta-carotene had a 22 percent reduced risk of heart ailments compared with women who consumed the least.

Researchers at the University of California, Los Angeles, found that men who consumed the most vitamin C had a 45 percent reduced risk of dying of heart disease; women had a 25 percent reduction in risk. The researchers used data from the first National Health and Nutrition Examination Survey, which included information about the vitamin intakes of more than 11,000 people.

Pumping Up HDL

The studies above did not specifically explore the relationship between blood cholesterol levels and antioxidants, but other research has examined the possibility that antioxidants may help raise HDL cholesterol and interfere with the oxidation of LDL.

"Several studies have shown that if you progress from consuming a relatively low amount of vitamin C—below 60 milligrams a day—up to about 200 to 300 milligrams a day, you'll experience a dose-related increase in HDL cholesterol," says Jeffrey Blumberg, Ph.D., chief of the Antioxidant Research Laboratory at the Jean Mayer USDA Human Nutrition Research Center on Aging at Tufts University in Boston. "This may account for some of the benefits of vitamin C in heart disease."

A study published by the New York Academy of Sciences in New York City, which compared the heart disease risks of 696 men and women ages 60 and over, found that consuming more than 180 milligrams of vitamin C a day—more than three times the DV—was associated with higher HDL cholesterol and lower blood pressure than consuming less than the DV of vitamin C a day. And at the Human Nutrition Research Center on Aging at Tufts, researchers found that higher blood levels of vitamin C (ascorbic acid) were associated with elevated HDL cholesterol and lower LDL cholesterol in more than 1,200 people.

Researchers at the University of California, San Diego, conducted two studies to determine the effects of vitamin E and beta-carotene—used individually, in combination and together with vitamin C—on the oxidation of LDL. In the first phase of the study, eight people consumed

60 milligrams of beta-carotene per day for three months. Then, for another three months, they added 1,600 international units of vitamin E a day to the beta-carotene. Finally, for another three months, the participants added 2,000 milligrams of vitamin C to the vitamin E and beta-carotene.

In the second phase of the study, the participants consumed only vitamin E supplements (1,600 international units a day) for five months. Researchers concluded that long-term use of vitamin E in high doses hindered the oxidation of LDL by 30 to 50 percent. Beta-carotene did not seem to affect LDL's resistance to oxidation.

The Great Debate: Food or Supplements?

Some researchers, including Dr. Blumberg, believe that the DVs— set at levels designed to prevent nutritional deficiencies—are too low to help fight disease. "Going by only the nutritional deficiency criteria, the DVs are absolutely correct," he says. "But if you ask 'How much vitamin C do I need to reduce my risk of heart disease, cancer or cataracts?' you'd get a much different answer than the DVs."

What's more, some people may find it difficult to even reach the DVs. In fact, a government survey found that just 9 percent of Americans eat the recommended minimum of five servings of fruits and vegetables a day. And it's difficult to consume potentially therapeutic amounts of some antioxidants through diet alone, say experts.

An important part of the answer, according to Dr. Blumberg, is antioxidant supplements. He recommends consuming between 250 and 1,000 milligrams of vitamin C and between 100 and 400 international units of vitamin E in supplement form. These doses are safe, he says. Since taking large amounts of vitamin C has been reported to cause diarrhea, however, and extremely high doses of vitamin E may cause headaches and diarrhea, be sure to check with your doctor before taking antioxidant supplements.

Because supplements can't compensate for bad dietary habits, it's crucial to follow a healthy diet rich in fruits, vegetables, whole grains, low-fat or nonfat dairy products and small amounts of meat, poultry and fish. "Rather than relying on supplements, eat foods rich in antioxidants," says Dr. Bersot. "They'll provide antioxidant vitamins as well as other nutritional substances that may be beneficial."

꩜

APPLES

Put the Crunch on Cholesterol

The next time you bite into a sweet, juicy McIntosh, consider this: Apples may very well help keep the doctor away—by lowering your blood cholesterol and protecting your heart.

The ingredient in apples that wallops blood cholesterol? Pectin, a sticky substance found in fruits and vegetables that works as a natural cholesterol cutter. "Pectin is a soluble fiber that helps draw cholesterol out of the system," says Audrey Cross, Ph.D., associate clinical professor at Columbia University's Institute of Human Nutrition in New York City. The average apple contains 1.08 grams of pectin.

Apples also contain flavonoids, certain chemicals that seem to short-circuit the process that leads "bad" LDL cholesterol to accumulate in the bloodstream. Dutch researchers who conducted a five-year study of 805 men ages 65 to 84 found that the men who ate the most flavonoids (also found in onions, tea and wine) were 50 percent less likely to have a first heart attack and die of heart disease than those who consumed the least.

You need to munch more than an apple a day to reap the full benefits of this fruit's power to clobber high cholesterol. But adding more apples and other high-fiber fruits and vegetables to your diet is a step in the right direction.

Scrubbing Clogged Arteries Clean

There's a wealth of evidence that points to apples' ability to help cut blood cholesterol. In a study conducted by David L. Gee, Ph.D., professor of food science and nutrition at Central Washington University in Ellensburg, 26 men with elevated cholesterol (ranging from 200 to 255 milligrams/deciliter) were divided into two groups. The first group ate three cookies with added apple fiber per day. These cookies contained a total of 14.5 grams of fiber, an amount equal to that found in four to five apples. The second group ate regular cookies. Otherwise, the men ate what they always ate.

After six weeks, in the group that ate the fiber-laden cookies, total cholesterol dropped an average of 15 points, or 7 percent. No improvements were seen in the placebo group.

In a follow-up study conducted by Dr. Gee and graduate student Karen Spencer, 25 men with cholesterol levels ranging from 200 to 270 milligrams/deciliter drank 20 ounces a day of FiberRich, a commercial apple juice brimming with pectin. After six weeks, the men's total cholesterol levels dipped an average of 10 percent, and their LDL cholesterol fell an average of 14 percent.

Other studies have pointed to apples' ability to lower blood cholesterol levels. In a French study, 30 healthy men and women added two to three apples to their diets each day for a month. Total cholesterol fell in 80 percent of the participants, by an average of 14 percent. One person's cholesterol plummeted 29 percent! HDL cholesterol, the "good" kind, rose slightly as well.

The Not-So-Forbidden Fruit

Perhaps the simplest way to take advantage of apples' power to pare blood cholesterol is to eat the raw fruit itself, say experts. "A fresh apple is a great snack food," says Evelyn Tribole, R.D., a dietitian in Beverly Hills, California, and author of *Healthy Homestyle Cooking*. But there are other ways to enjoy the delicious taste of apples. Try these suggestions.

• Mix sliced apples with a low-fat cheese, sprinkle with fresh chives and serve on romaine lettuce. You might also toss sliced apples with raisins, almonds and cooked chicken and splash the salad with tarragon vinegar.

• Add apples to baked goods. "You can grate apples into almost anything that you bake, including low-fat muffins and cakes," says Tribole. Try grating one large apple into a recipe that yields six large muffins.

• Sauté a side dish. Sautéed apples are a delicious accompaniment to meat (preferably leaner cuts). After sautéing turkey cutlets, for example, remove the meat from the pan and add sliced peeled apples to the meat juices. Sauté the apples for five minutes, then stir in $\frac{1}{2}$ cup of apple juice and cook until the apples are soft (about three minutes). Serve with the cutlets.

Heart-Healthy ♡
Indulgences

APPLE PIE: A DELICIOUS WAY TO BENEFIT FROM PECTIN

A lot of evidence suggests that apples can help cut blood cholesterol, thanks to a sticky substance called pectin. Found in some fruits and vegetables, pectin is a soluble fiber that's thought to draw cholesterol out of the system. But apples are also full of flavonoids, which are the chemicals that appear to block the process that allows harmful LDL cholesterol to clog up your arteries.

So help yourself to a slice of apple pie every now and then. Just be sure to leave some of the crust on your plate—it's loaded with shortening, a hydrogenated fat that's bad for your arteries.

If you want to cut the fat in your homemade piecrust, here are some tips.

Use less shortening. Although many pastry recipes tend to be fairly exact, it is often possible to cut the amount of shortening by about one-third without having a big impact on the texture of the crust.

Replace it with oil. If you use canola or safflower oil in place of some of the solid shortening, you'll be exchanging some of the saturated fat for a more heart-healthy monounsaturated or polyunsaturated fat.

• Bake a guilt-free pastry. Chop up some apples, add cinnamon and a little sugar, wrap the apples in phyllo dough and bake, suggests Tribole. "You'll end up with something like apple strudel that's very low in fat," she says.

As healthful as apples are, you can sabotage their goodness. "Consuming apples in a pie with a thick crust loaded with butter isn't the best way of eating them," says Sheah Rarback, R.D., director of nutrition at the University of Miami School of Medicine's Mailman Center. You can indulge your sweet tooth occasionally, says Rarback. But if you want to help lower your blood cholesterol, it's best to munch fresh apples or to prepare them in some other healthy way, she says.

To keep apples crisp, wrap them in a plastic bag and store them in the refrigerator. Apples kept at room temperature soften ten times faster than refrigerated fruit.

~❊~

ARGININE

A Cholesterol Fighter in Snack Form

You probably "take" this possible cholesterol fighter right now without even knowing it. It's arginine, an amino acid found in chicken and all other meats as well as in plant foods such as nuts. The average person eats about 5 grams of it daily.

Your body transforms arginine into a natural substance called nitric oxide, the most potent blood vessel relaxer known. Preliminary research suggests that an extra 6 to 9 milligrams of arginine a day, which may improve coronary blood flow, can help lower cholesterol levels. How? By acting as an antioxidant and also by keeping blood vessels elastic so that blood flow is improved and cholesterol deposits are reduced.

The connection between arginine and heart health has not been conclusively shown, however. Robert Eckel, M.D., a former chairman of the nutrition committee for the American Heart Association and professor of medicine at the University of Colorado Center for Human Nutrition in Denver, calls the evidence for arginine a work in progress.

Nevertheless, researcher John Cooke, M.D., associate professor of medicine and director of the vascular section at Stanford University, argues in favor of arginine for certain people.

According to Dr. Cooke, you may want to think about arginine if you're an exerciser with heart or artery disease, since the amino acid may help with blood-flow problems. If this is your situation, it's definitely best to check with your doctor before starting any exercise program or using this supplement. For people with impaired blood flow to the heart or legs, Dr. Cooke says that those with high cholesterol are most likely to benefit from arginine; people with diabetes and high blood pressure are less likely to respond to it.

Dr. Cooke helped develop HeartBars, which are one of the two sources of arginine other than food. Marketed as a dietary therapy for people with cardiovascular disease, each bar has 180 calories. Eating two a day supplies more than 6 milligrams of arginine as well as other heart-healthy nutrients such as niacin and soy protein.

Arginine is also available in capsules. While they are convenient and easy to swallow, you'd have to take 6 to 18 capsules a day to get the same amount of arginine as in a HeartBar.

Whether you're using HeartBars or capsules, experts say it's a good idea to split your daily dose of arginine into two or three equal doses taken at different times of the day to maintain even levels in your blood (provided, of course, that your doctor has given you the go-ahead to use the supplements).

ঌৠৈ

ARTICHOKES

Newcomers to the Cholesterol Wars

Artichokes are a springtime staple, but research now shows that they can have year-round benefits.

German researchers gave 143 men and women who had high levels of total cholesterol (more than 280 milligrams/deciliter) either 1,800 milligrams of dried artichoke extract or a placebo (inactive pill) every day for six weeks. By the study's end, those who took the extract lowered their cholesterol by an average of 18 percent. The placebo group's cholesterol dropped by about 8 percent. In addition, the researchers found that levels of "bad" LDL cholesterol fell more than 20 percent in the people who took the extract and that their ratio of protective HDL to LDL also improved.

How does this extract help "choke" cholesterol? Artichokes contain a compound called cynarin, which increases production of bile by the liver. Studies also show that the extract boosts the flow of bile from the gallbladder. Bile plays a key role in the excretion of excess cholesterol from the body.

Even better, there were no drug-related side effects reported during the study. The researchers think that indicates that someday, artichoke extract may be widely used—at any time of year.

Meanwhile, you can team artichokes with other vegetables to create a side dish that can help you reap the cholesterol-cutting benefits and taste of artichokes plus the heart-healthy benefits of olive oil.

GREEN BEANS WITH PEPPERS AND ARTICHOKES

MAKES 4 SERVINGS

12 ounces small red potatoes
8 ounces green beans
1 cup chopped roasted red bell peppers
8 water-packed artichoke hearts, halved
⅓ cup tarragon vinegar
1 tablespoon olive oil
1 teaspoon Dijon mustard
1 clove garlic, minced
½ teaspoon dried marjoram
¼ teaspoon ground black pepper
¼ teaspoon Worcestershire sauce

In a large saucepan, bring 1" of water to a boil. Place the potatoes on a steaming rack and set the rack in the pan. Cover and steam for 15 minutes, or until tender. Set aside to cool. When the potatoes are cool enough to handle, slice thinly and place in a large bowl.

In a medium saucepan, blanch the beans in boiling water for 5 minutes. Drain and add to the potatoes. Add the peppers and artichokes and toss to combine.

In a small bowl, whisk together the vinegar, oil, mustard, garlic, marjoram, black pepper, and Worcestershire sauce. Pour over the vegetables and toss to combine.

PER SERVING: 172 CALORIES, 5.8 G FAT (30% OF CALORIES), 3.7 G PROTEIN, 30.5 G CARBOHYDRATES, 0 MG CHOLESTEROL, 2.1 G DIETARY FIBER, 113 MG SODIUM

AVOCADOS

This "Fat" Fruit Fights Cholesterol

Fattening. Oil-soaked. Hell on the waistline.

If you're like many people, you might use epithets like these to describe the otherwise tasty avocado. But hold the name-calling for a second. If you're trying to lower your blood cholesterol, you may want to indulge in this green fruit once in a while: Avocados are high in monounsaturated fat, which is known to reduce LDL, or "bad," cholesterol. Avocados are especially rich in oleic acid, the same cholesterol-busting monounsaturate found in olive and canola oils.

The only catch: Avocados are extremely high in fat. And consuming too much of any fat, even monounsaturated fat, isn't a good idea, say experts. Eaten sparingly, however, avocados just might help you chip a few points off your cholesterol count—deliciously.

Going Down, Down, Down

The connection between avocados and lower blood cholesterol began with a hunch: A team of Australian researchers suspected the link and decided to test their theory. In this study, 15 women alternated between a low-fat, high-carbohydrate diet (21 percent fat calories) and an avocado-enriched diet (36 percent fat calories) in which they ate from $\frac{1}{2}$ to $1\frac{1}{2}$ avocados per day.

After three weeks on the avocado-rich diet, the women's total cholesterol fell from an average of 236 to 217 milligrams/deciliter, or 8.2 percent, compared with 4.9 percent after three weeks on the low-fat plan. More significantly, however, "good" HDL cholesterol plummeted an average of 14 percent on the low-fat plan and not at all on the avocado diet. As a result, the ratio of total cholesterol to HDL increased 10.4 percent in the women on the low-fat plan but decreased 14.9 percent in the avocado-eaters.

Avocados may also be a dietary asset for people with non-insulin-dependent (type 2) diabetes, for whom consuming too many carbohydrates can cause triglyceride and blood sugar problems. A Mexican study found that partially replacing carbohydrates with monounsaturated fat lowered triglycerides in 16 women with type 2 diabetes. In this study, the women ate a baseline diet for one month. They then alternated between two diets. The first diet was high in monounsaturated fat (40 percent total fat calories), derived primarily from avocados. The second food plan was high in complex carbohydrates (20 percent total fat calories).

Both diets lowered the women's total cholesterol slightly. But their triglycerides fell 20 percent on the avocado-enriched diet, compared with 7 percent on the high-carbohydrate plan. The women's blood sugar levels were not affected by either diet.

Get Monos in Moderation

Avocados contain zero dietary cholesterol, which is found only in animal-derived foods such as eggs, milk and meats. But don't gobble avocados with abandon: From 71 to 88 percent of this fruit's calories come from fat. "Using one-eighth of an average avocado in a salad adds about five grams of fat," says Janet Lepke, R.D., a dietitian in Santa Monica, California, and a spokesperson for the American Dietetic Association.

Most people don't eat more than half of an avocado at a time, however. "You shouldn't consume too much of any fat, saturated or unsaturated," says Wahida Karmally, R.D., director of nutrition at the Irving Center for Clinical Research at Columbia-Presbyterian Medical Center in New York City and a member of the American Heart Association's nutrition committee. So substitute avocados for foods high in saturated fat rather than add avocados to an already high-fat diet, recommends Karmally.

A Little Goes a Long Way

Many people stud their salads with chunks of avocado or add a few slices of the fruit to a sandwich. But you might try these serving suggestions, too.

• Try topping your baked potato with mashed avocado, suggests the California Avocado Commission. A tablespoon of butter contains 100 calories, mostly from saturated fat. A tablespoon of mashed avocado, on the other hand, contains 20 calories, mostly from monounsaturated fat.

• To perk up baked chicken, "top it with slices of avocado before serving," suggests Tammy Baker, R.D., a nutritionist in Cave Creek, Arizona, and a spokesperson for the American Dietetic Association.

• The next time you make potato salad, use less mayonnaise and add some mashed avocado instead. You'll consume less saturated fat and dietary cholesterol and more heart-healthy monounsaturated fat.

• Slice an avocado in half, remove the seed and stuff the fruit with chicken, seafood or pasta salad prepared with low-fat or cholesterol-free mayo. To keep the avocado from turning brown, rub the flesh with a little lemon juice.

Note: If you buy avocados that aren't yet ripe enough to eat, you can speed up the ripening process by putting them in a paper bag and setting them aside for a few days.

BEANS

The Core of Heart-Smart Cuisine

Think the bean is peasant food? Think again. The formerly humble legume has become hot stuff, especially among folks who want a high-protein, low-fat and inexpensive alternative to red meat.

What's more, beans can help deal a knockout blow to elevated cholesterol: Many varieties are loaded with soluble fiber, which has been proven to help lower cholesterol. "Beans also contain omega-3 fatty acids and loads of calcium," says Neal Barnard, M.D., president of the Physicians Committee for Responsible Medicine in Washington, D.C.

CAN'T BEAT THESE BEANS

Want to add fiber power to your cholesterol-lowering diet? Load up on these legumes.

LEGUME (½ CUP COOKED)	SOLUBLE FIBER (G)
Kidney beans	2.8
Cranberry beans	2.7
Lima beans	2.7
Black beans	2.4
Navy beans	2.2
Lentils	2.0
Pinto beans	1.9
Great Northern beans	1.4
Chickpeas	1.3
Split peas	1.1

Omega-3 fatty acids, also found in certain fatty fish, are a type of polyunsaturated fat, which helps prevent cardiovascular disease.

Beans' nutritional pedigree and culinary versatility mean they're perfect in virtually any dish, from fiery chili to savory soups. Best of all, whipping up quick, healthy bean dishes can be as simple as opening a can. Want more good reasons to pile your plate with beans? Read on.

At the University of Kentucky in Lexington, James W. Anderson, M.D., professor of medicine and clinical nutrition in the university's College of Medicine and author of *Dr. Anderson's High-Fiber Fitness Plan*, and his colleagues instructed 20 men with cholesterol levels exceeding 260 milligrams/deciliter to eat about 1½ cups total of pinto and navy beans a day. After three weeks, the men's total cholesterol fell an average of 56 points, while their "bad" LDL cholesterol plunged 51 points.

And in another study led by Dr. Anderson, 28 men with high cholesterol ate one eight-ounce can of beans in tomato sauce every day for three weeks. The men's total cholesterol dropped 10.4 percent, and their triglyceride levels declined 10.8 percent.

Researchers in New Zealand put 40 people with high cholesterol on a low-fat diet to which either cooked beans or oat bran was added.

These folks' total cholesterol declined slightly on both diets. But their "good" HDL cholesterol rose significantly when they ate the beans rather than the oat bran.

The Basics of Bean Cookery

Beans warrant a prominent place on a cholesterol-lowering menu. These tips can get you started.

• If you want to use dried whole beans, you'll need to soak them. Soak the beans in cold water overnight, so they'll be ready to cook the next day. Or try the quick soak method: Boil the beans for two minutes, then set them aside to soak for an hour or so.

• To bypass soaking or quick soaking altogether, opt for lentils and split peas, suggests Dr. Anderson. These legumes don't require soaking and cook up in a fraction of the time of dried beans. "While split peas and lentils are a little lower in fiber than the beans we used in our studies, they should still help lower cholesterol," says Dr. Anderson.

• Add canned beans to soups, salads and casseroles, suggests Dr. Anderson. Rinse the beans to remove excess sodium.

• To give stews a fiber boost, add a can of chickpeas, kidney beans, lima beans or black beans.

• Enjoy burritos made with beans instead of beef, suggests Dr. Barnard. "There's nothing better than a homemade bean burrito with jalapeño peppers," he says. Try topping your burrito with low-fat or fat-free cheese and a dab of fat-free sour cream.

• Mix any type of mashed canned beans with chopped onions, fresh garlic and low-sodium tamari (a kind of soy sauce), suggests Michael Klaper, M.D., health director of the Royal Atlantic Health Spa in Pompano Beach, Florida, and author of *Vegan Nutrition: Pure and Simple*. Spread the mixture on crackers or spoon into taco shells.

• Add a trickle of olive oil and some fresh garlic to mashed canned chickpeas and spread on your favorite bread, suggests Dr. Klaper.

• Explore the ways different cultures use beans. You might try making a spicy Cuban black bean soup; Middle Eastern hummus (a savory spread of chickpeas, lemon juice, garlic and fresh mint, served with pita bread); Italian *pasta e fagioli* (pasta with beans); or Southern-style hoppin' John (black-eyed peas and rice—hold the ham).

• If you're dining in a Mexican restaurant, avoid refried beans, says Martin Yadrick, R.D., a dietitian in Manhattan Beach, California, and a spokesperson for the American Dietetic Association. "Traditional refried beans are prepared with lard," he says. "Ask for pinto beans or black beans, which contain a minimal amount of fat."

Degassing Legumes

Beans can cause gastrointestinal distress in some people. The gas-producing culprits: stachyose and raffinose, sugars that are the by-products of beans, says Linda Van Horn, R.D., Ph.D., associate professor of preventive medicine at Northwestern University Medical School in Chicago. To help prevent gas, "soak beans before you cook them and discard the water they've been soaking in," advises Dr. Van Horn. "Soaking beans breaks down some of these sugars."

You might also consider trying a product called Beano. This over-the-counter product really does help reduce gas in some people, according to a study conducted at the University of California, San Diego. Folks who consumed eight drops of Beano after the first bite of a meal of meatless chili seemed to experience fewer gas eruptions than those who had taken a placebo, according to the participants' self-reported symptoms.

∼❀∽

CALCIUM

The Multi-Talented Mineral

Drink your milk! It's good for growing bones."

As a kid, you probably heard this maternal refrain hundreds of times. And Mom was right: Milk—or rather the calcium in milk—does help build strong bones. Calcium is also the first line of defense against osteoporosis, the crippling bone-thinning disease that afflicts about 24 million people, mostly women, over age 65.

But along with fracture-proofing your bones, calcium might also help protect your ticker: Some studies indicate that calcium may play a role in lowering blood cholesterol. While the jury is still out on this theory, the evidence is intriguing. Read on.

How Calcium Licks LDL

Heart disease experts have suspected since the 1950s that calcium might lower cholesterol. But most of their studies, while promising, have yielded less than sensational results. That's because most of the early research focused on the effects of calcium on total cholesterol. More recent studies have analyzed calcium's effects on the separate components of total cholesterol, LDL (the "bad" kind) and HDL (the "good" kind), which experts consider more sensitive measures of heart disease risk. And the news is encouraging.

Researchers at the University of Texas Southwestern Medical Center at Dallas, headed by Margo Denke, M.D., associate professor of medicine in the Center for Human Nutrition, put 13 men with moderately high cholesterol on either a high-calcium diet (2,200 milligrams of calcium per day) or a low-calcium diet (410 milligrams of calcium per day) for ten weeks. For the next ten weeks, the men resumed their regular diets. During the study's final ten weeks, the men who first consumed the high-calcium diet followed the low-calcium plan, and vice versa.

The researchers found that the men's total cholesterol fell an average of 6 percent on the high-calcium diet. Even more significantly, their LDL cholesterol dropped an average of 11 percent. Since experts generally agree that every 1 percent decrease in LDL cholesterol results in a 2 percent decrease in heart disease risk, the participants' risk dropped over 20 percent.

In another study, researchers at the Hennepin County Medical Center in Minneapolis had 56 men and women with mildly to moderately high blood cholesterol follow a low-fat diet and consume 1,200 milligrams of calcium a day. These folks' LDL cholesterol dropped 4.4 percent, which theoretically decreased their heart disease risk by nearly 10 percent. What's more, their HDL cholesterol increased 4.1 percent.

How might calcium reduce cholesterol? According to the University of Texas study, calcium may both block the absorption of saturated fat and bind with cholesterol-containing bile acids in the digestive system. The body then excretes these acids, giving excess cholesterol the boot, too. In fact, the men in the University of Texas study excreted 13 percent saturated fat while following the high-calcium diet, compared with only 6 percent while on the low-calcium plan.

Fat-Free Ways to Bone Up Your Diet

Whether the link between increased calcium consumption and lower blood cholesterol will be borne out by further study remains to be seen. Still, "there are many good reasons to increase your calcium intake," says Robert Heaney, M.D., professor of medicine at Creighton University School of Medicine in Omaha, Nebraska, and an expert on calcium.

The most crucial reason? Many people simply don't get enough of this vital mineral. The optimum intake is 1,000 milligrams a day for women ages 25 to 50, menopausal women (ages 51 to 65) who take estrogen and men ages 25 to 65. That amount jumps to 1,500 milligrams a day for menopausal women who don't take estrogen and for all men and women over age 65. Yet it's estimated that 50 percent of women over age 35 consume less than 500 milligrams of calcium a day—far less than they need.

Fortunately, it's easy to fortify your heart and bones with calcium. Simply eat more low-fat or fat-free milk, yogurt and cheese, which contain all of the calcium of whole milk dairy products with much less of the artery-plugging saturated fat. Other good sources of calcium include sardines and canned salmon, calcium-fortified orange juice and green vegetables, particularly bok choy and kale.

Choosing a Supplement

If you suspect that you're not getting enough calcium through your diet, you might consider taking calcium supplements, available in drugstores and health food stores, says Dr. Heaney. The most common supplements contain calcium carbonate.

The following guidelines can help you choose calcium supplements properly, says Dr. Heaney.

• Take calcium supplements in small doses—500 milligrams or less at a time.

• Take calcium carbonate supplements with meals to ensure good

CALCULATE YOUR CALCIUM QUOTA

Chances are you won't find a single-dose multivitamin/mineral supplement that contains 100 percent of the optimal amount of 1,000 milligrams of calcium. And if you're a woman over age 50 or a man over age 65, you need even more calcium: 1,500 milligrams per day (150 percent of the Daily Value). So you may want to consider taking a calcium supplement. Here's how to find out if you're giving your heart and bones a steady supply of this essential nutrient.

1. Determine your calcium goal.
2. Subtract 300 milligrams for each serving of milk, yogurt, cheese or calcium-fortified orange juice that you typically consume each day.
3. Subtract any calcium that you may get from a multivitamin/mineral supplement. Most supplements contain 200 milligrams or less.

If, after your calculations, you're coming up short of your calcium goal, you need to take a calcium supplement, says William P. Castelli, M.D., medical director of the Framingham Cardiovascular Institute, a wellness program at Metro West Medical Center in Massachusetts.

absorption, says Dr. Heaney. He recommends chewable supplements: "They disintegrate best," he says. Avoid "natural source" calcium carbonate supplements made from bonemeal, dolomite or oyster shell, however. Some studies indicate that these products may contain unhealthy amounts of lead.

• Limit your intake of fatty foods, caffeine, alcohol and tobacco products. All can hinder calcium absorption.

• Make sure to get the Daily Value of vitamin D (400 international units): It's essential for calcium absorption. Eat foods fortified with vitamin D, including fat-free milk and some breads and cereals. Or consider taking a daily multivitamin/mineral supplement that meets 100 percent of your daily vitamin D requirement.

• Try to avoid calcium supplements that contain aluminum. This chemical can deplete the body's supply of phosphate, which it needs to absorb calcium, says Dr. Heaney. "But if you have a peptic ulcer and need to take supplements that contain aluminum, make sure you get extra calcium," he advises.

• Don't take calcium supplements with high-fiber wheat bran cereals: These cereals can reduce calcium absorption by 25 percent.

• Drink lots of water to help avoid constipation, a possible side effect of calcium supplements.

Supplements are not a substitute for a low-fat diet or cholesterol-lowering drugs (if your doctor has prescribed them), says Dr. Denke. But "if you're eating a low-fat, low–saturated fat, low-cholesterol diet, some additional calcium may be helpful," she says. "Women might want an extra 1,000 milligrams a day of calcium—it can also help protect against osteoporosis." For men, taking an additional 800 milligrams of calcium over the optimal amounts may be sufficient, she says.

While research indicates that calcium does not heighten the risk of kidney stone formation, if you have kidney stones, it's still a good idea to check with your doctor before taking calcium supplements. In fact, says Dr. Heaney, "a high-calcium diet may protect against the absorption of oxalic acid, the principal risk factor in the formation of kidney stones."

CANOLA OIL

The Lightest of All

Safflower and corn oils, which are high in polyunsaturated fat, can lower "bad" LDL cholesterol. But there's a trade-off: Polyunsaturated fat can cause "good" HDL cholesterol to slide, too. And coconut and palm kernel oils (the so-called tropical oils) are brimming with saturated fat, which can launch your blood cholesterol into an upward trajectory and stop up your coronary arteries.

Enter canola oil. This super oil can lower LDL cholesterol while it maintains or even raises HDL cholesterol. That's because canola oil is high in monounsaturated fat, the kind associated with reducing blood cholesterol.

Promising Results

A number of studies have shown that canola oil can be effective in reducing elevated cholesterol. For example, at the Kenneth L. Jordan Heart Foundation and Research Center in Montclair, New Jersey, and Elmhurst General Hospital in Queens, New York, 36 people with either high blood cholesterol or high blood pressure added one ounce (about two tablespoons) of canola oil to their diets per day, using it in place of other oils and spreads. After four months, the participants' average total cholesterol fell from 254 to 248 milligrams/deciliter, and their LDL cholesterol dipped from 173 to 160 milligrams/deciliter. What's more, these folks' HDL cholesterol rose slightly, from 47 to 51 milligrams/deciliter.

Researchers at the University of Helsinki in Finland compared the effect on blood cholesterol of a diet high in monounsaturated fat and a diet high in polyunsaturated fat. For two weeks, the researchers fed 59 people a baseline diet that was high in saturated fat. Then the participants alternated between two diets—the first enriched with canola oil, and the second, with sunflower oil. Both diets supplied 38 percent of calories from fat. But the sunflower oil diet was higher in polyunsaturated fat and lower in monounsaturated fat.

After 25 days on each diet, total cholesterol among men and women on the canola-enriched diet dropped 15 percent, and LDL cholesterol levels dipped 23 percent below the baseline level. By comparision, the total cholesterol of the sunflower oil group decreased 12 percent, and the LDL cholesterol fell 17 percent from the baseline. Neither diet affected levels of HDL cholesterol.

What about Olive Oil?

How does canola oil fare against olive oil, also touted for its ability to slash LDL while it maintains or even raises HDL cholesterol?

Canola oil and olive oil have virtually the same effect on blood cholesterol, says Alice H. Lichtenstein, D.Sc., assistant professor of nutrition at Tufts University in Medford, Massachusetts, and a scientist at the Jean Mayer USDA Human Nutrition Research Center on Aging in Boston. "The effects on LDL cholesterol are comparable," says Dr. Lichtenstein. "No one is saying that there's an advantage to using olive oil over canola oil, or vice versa."

And while canola oil is lower in monounsaturated fat than olive oil, it is also lower in saturated fat. "Of the five vegetable oils lowest in saturated fat—canola, olive, corn, safflower and sunflower—none is lower than canola," says Evelyn Tribole, R.D., a dietitian in Beverly Hills, California, and author of *Healthy Homestyle Cooking.* "Canola oil contains 6 percent saturated fat, and olive oil 15 percent saturated fat."

The bottom line? You can use both canola oil and olive oil as part of a heart-healthy diet. The best course of action, advises Tribole, is to replace the saturated fat in your diet, such as butter, with unsaturated fat, such as canola oil.

Salads, No—Popcorn, Yes

Unlike olive oil, canola oil doesn't have a pronounced flavor. But that's not necessarily a disadvantage, especially if you don't enjoy the robust flavor of olive oil.

In fact, canola oil's subtle flavor can be a plus—it's a natural choice for some dishes. "You can use canola oil in place of safflower or corn oil," says Tammy Baker, R.D., a nutritionist in Cave Creek, Arizona, and a spokesperson for the American Dietetic Association. Try substituting canola oil for butter when you're sautéing vegetables or in baked goods and sauces, suggests Baker, or when you're making popcorn. When not to use canola oil, says Baker: in salad dressings. It's way too bland to add flavor to your fixin's.

However you decide to use canola oil, keep it fresh. Oils high in monounsaturated fat tend to go bad faster than other oils. So if you haven't used up a bottle of canola oil about a month after opening it, store it in the refrigerator.

⊱✿⊰

CARROTS

Fight Cholesterol with Fiber Power

Crisp and crunchy, carrots may well qualify as the ultimate healthy snack. They're brimming with beta-carotene and vitamin C— antioxidant nutrients believed to help protect against a variety of ailments, including cancer—as well as with vitamin A. What's more, these sweet, crunchy veggies are packed with soluble fiber, the kind proven to help deflate blood cholesterol.

More specifically, carrots are rich in calcium pectate, a certain type of soluble fiber that may bestow special cholesterol-lowering power, according to Peter D. Hoagland, Ph.D., a research chemist for the USDA. Dr. Hoagland's research indicates that calcium pectate helps to bind bile acids, the substances that assist in the digestion of fats and in the transportation of cholesterol out of the body.

A study conducted outside the United States seems to back Dr. Hoagland's research. Scientists at Western General Hospital in Edinburgh, Scotland, had five people eat 200 grams of raw carrots (about two carrots) each morning. After three weeks of this morning ritual, the people's cholesterol levels fell 11 percent. And their cholesterol remained lowered for another three weeks after they stopped eating the daily carrots.

Cooked carrots appear to help lower cholesterol just as well as raw carrots, says Dr. Hoagland. "The fiber in cooked carrots seems to have the same ability to bind bile acids as the fiber in raw carrots," he says. "Calcium pectate still ends up in the gut, where it can interact with bile acids."

Here's how to add more carrots to your diet.

• Make sure carrots are fresh. If you're buying them by the bunch, choose the ones with the freshest-looking tops: The fresher the greens, the fresher the carrots, says Mindy Hermann, R.D., a nutrition consultant in Mount Kisco, New York. "If you buy bagged carrots, feel the vegetables through the bag and avoid those that feel flabby or rubbery," says Hermann.

• Many experts suggest steaming carrots to preserve their nutrients. Boiling carrots drains 50 percent of their beta-carotene and 90 percent of their vitamin C.

• Try snacking on prewashed, prepeeled baby carrots. "Try them with a fat-free dip—fat-free sour cream or yogurt mixed with a dry dip mix," says Evelyn Tribole, R.D., a dietitian in Beverly Hills, California, and author of *Healthy Homestyle Cooking*.

• Want to make a dish bursting with fiber and antioxidant vitamins? "Make a sweet-potato-and-carrot casserole, and season it with a little ginger or nutmeg," suggests Mona Sutnick, R.D., Ed.D., a dietitian in Philadelphia and a spokesperson for the American Dietetic Association.

• Make roasted carrots, suggests Barbie Casselman, a nutrition consultant in Toronto. Here's how: Spray sliced carrots with nonstick cooking spray, arrange them on a nonstick baking sheet and bake at 425° for 20 to 25 minutes. "When you make carrots this way, no one misses the cream sauce," says Casselman.

CHICKEN

A Decent Choice Made Better

For years, the ultimate in fine dining was a nice, thick, juicy steak. But when doctors started telling us what consuming too much fatty red meat could do to our coronary arteries—and to our hearts—many of us modified our carnivorous ways and started eating more chicken.

"Generally speaking, chicken contains less saturated fat and more polyunsaturated fat than beef," says Gene A. Spiller, D.Sc., Ph.D., director of the Health Research and Studies Center in Los Altos, California, and author of *The Superpyramid Eating Program*. Three ounces of lean, broiled filet mignon contains 8.5 grams of fat, 3.2 grams of it saturated. The same amount of skinless chicken breast contains 3.1 grams of fat and less than 1 gram of saturated fat.

But hold on. While eating plates of red meat the size of Idaho isn't a good idea, all red meat isn't necessarily bad for you, say experts. Nor is all chicken necessarily good for you: If you're trying to lower your blood cholesterol, eating three or four pieces of fried chicken is definitely not what the doctor ordered.

To make poultry a part of a heart-healthy diet, say experts, you need to choose the right cuts of chicken and prepare them with little or no fat. "Think lean when you put chicken on your table," says Dr. Spiller.

Poultry Pointers

These suggestions can help you trim the fat—and a significant number of calories—from chicken.

• Buy the leanest birds. Broilers and fryers are lower in fat than roasters.

• Bake, broil or roast chicken. These cooking methods allow the fat to drip off the bird. Frying chicken, on the other hand, adds fat and calories.

• Eat "light." The white meat portions of a chicken contain less fat than the dark meat, and the breast is the leanest part of the bird: Three ounces of skinless chicken breast gets 19 percent of its calories from fat, while a whole skinless chicken leg—thigh and drumstick— gets a whopping 40 percent of its calories from fat.

• If you can't resist dark meat, eat smaller amounts of it less often, suggests Susan Kleiner, R.D., Ph.D., a nutritionist in Seattle and author of *The High-Performance Cookbook*. While a thigh or drumstick contains more fat than a breast, "dark meat still contains less fat than most beef, relatively speaking," says Dr. Kleiner.

• Coat a pan or wok with fat-free cooking spray and stir-fry chicken with fresh or frozen vegetables, herbs and spices.

• Microwave skinless chicken breasts and top them with salsa, low-fat spaghetti sauce or lemon-pepper seasoning. (Make sure the chicken is cooked thoroughly.)

Heart-Healthy♡
Indulgences

CHICKEN FAJITAS: FOR A MEXICAN MEAL MAKEOVER

Prepared with heart-healthy ingredients, chicken fajitas—a mainstay of Mexican cuisine—can help clobber cholesterol. Here's how to get the benefits.

Sauté strips of chicken breast with red and green bell peppers, onions and tomatoes in a teaspoon of oil, then fold the mixture in a corn tortilla. For variety, use cholesterol-fighting vegetables like broccoli and mushrooms.

It's thought that fajitas originated with cowboys in southwestern Texas. If you want to be totally traditional, you can use beef instead of chicken. (The word *fajita* is the diminutive form of *faja*, Spanish for the "little belt" of skirt steak just behind the front leg of a steer.) For the heart-healthiest effects, use lean flank steak or beef tenderloin.

• Pass up fast-food fried chicken, which is loaded with sodium, fat and cholesterol. But if you must indulge, stem the damage: Eat one or two pieces of chicken and fill up on vegetables, rice, a baked potato or a salad with low-fat or fat-free dressing, advises Mary Donkersloot, R.D., a dietitian in Beverly Hills, California, a spokesperson for the California Dietetic Association and author of *The Fast Food Diet.*

• Better yet, make your own "fried" chicken in the oven, suggests Evelyn Tribole, R.D., a dietitian in Beverly Hills, California, in her book *Healthy Homestyle Cooking*: Coat skinless chicken breasts with egg whites (not the yolks), a small amount of flour and cornflake crumbs and bake at 375°.

To Skin or Not to Skin

If you consider the crispy, crunchy skin the best part of the chicken, being told not to indulge may leave you feeling deprived. So if you know you're not going to give up the skin, at least practice damage control.

"If you insist on leaving the skin on, you definitely shouldn't fry the chicken, which will add more fat," says Bettye Nowlin, R.D., a dietitian in Los Angeles and a spokesperson for the American Dietetic Association. "Instead, you should roast or broil your chicken, keep your portion size small and avoid high-fat foods for the rest of the day."

If you're serious about reducing your intake of dietary fat, however, it's best to avoid the skin altogether, says William P. Castelli, M.D., medical director of the Framingham Cardiovascular Institute, a wellness program at Metro West Medical Center in Massachusetts. "Take off the skin and toss it out!" he says. Think of it this way: By stripping off the skin, you'll slash your intake of saturated fat in half and save yourself some calories in the bargain.

There is some good news about chicken skin, however: Despite what you may think, you don't have to remove the skin before you cook chicken. Researchers at the University of Minnesota found that removing the skin after cooking rather than beforehand doesn't affect the fat content of the meat. "The fat that's in the skin stays there—it doesn't migrate into the meat," says dietitian Linda Dieleman, R.D., of the University of Minnesota Inter-College Nutrition Consortium in St. Paul.

As a bonus, "leaving the skin on during baking will help keep the chicken moist," says Lisa Lauri, R.D., nutrition consultant at North Shore University Hospital in Manhasset, New York.

CHILE PEPPERS

Fire Up Your Blood Fats

For some thrill-seeking folks, eating chile peppers is as exhilarating as skydiving or rock climbing. Eyes streaming, noses leaking, these self-proclaimed fire-eaters—who call riding the wave of chile pepper heat mouth surfing—enjoy setting their tongues ablaze. And they never seem to run out of ways to send their mouths into meltdown: Chile aficionados add their favorite pepper to soups, stews, salsas and sauces, roast them and stuff them with cheese, even add them to ice cream.

But those with flame-resistant gullets may actually reap some health benefits from chile peppers. These pungent peppers are high in vitamin A, which is thought to boost immunity and protect against cancer, and vitamin C, which may help deflate blood pressure. Even more significantly, capsaicin—the substance that gives chile peppers their bite— may also help lower triglycerides, a type of blood fat implicated in heart disease. Chile peppers may even reduce the risk of heart attack and stroke by increasing the blood's ability to break up dangerous clots.

It appears that capsaicin (also used to relieve psoriasis and arthritis pain) may impact more on triglycerides than on cholesterol. But the few studies that have explored the connection between capsaicin and blood fats have yielded intriguing results. When researchers in India fed capsaicin to laboratory rats along with their normal diet, for example, the rodents' triglyceride levels fell, although their cholesterol levels weren't affected. Researchers at the Ohio State University College of Medicine in Columbus also administered capsaicin to rats; these rodents' triglycerides fell as well.

The best news of all? Despite chile peppers' fearsome reputation, it's entirely possible to enjoy their three-alarm flavor without losing taste buds in the process. You just have to know how to handle the heat—and proceed with caution. Here's how.

Small Peppers Pack Big Heat

There are over 100 kinds of chile pepper, and they're available in a variety of forms, including fresh, dried and powdered. But when it comes to generating heat, not all chiles are created equal.

You can't always judge a chile pepper's heat by its size or color. Generally speaking, the smaller the pepper, the hotter it is: Small, narrow chile peppers, including the cayenne and serrano, pack more capsaicin than larger, milder peppers, such as the poblano and Anaheim.

The jalapeño pepper is one of the most popular chiles in the United States. But while most people consider this plump, bright red or dark green pepper a real stinger, its heat pales in comparison with that of the habañero, the most blistering chile of all.

It's the hottest pepper on record," says Dave DeWitt, author of *The*

Heart-Healthy ♡
Indulgences

JALAPEÑO ICE CREAM: TANTALIZE YOUR TASTE BUDS AND REDUCE TRIGLYCERIDES

Perhaps you've seen it on the menu at upscale restaurants: jalapeño ice cream. Think it sounds way out? Give it a try. You may find that the unusual combination—sweet, cold and spicy hot—is quite tasty. As a bonus, capsaicin, the substance that gives chile peppers their bite, may help lower triglycerides, a type of blood fat that has been implicated in heart disease.

To make your own version of this trendy treat, puree a chile pepper and add a little to your evening dish of low-fat or fat-free ice cream. Vanilla is a good choice for your first taste test, but chocolate works well, too.

Whole Chile Pepper Book. A measurement called the Scoville unit is used to determine the heat of chile peppers, he explains. While the jalapeño pepper averages about 5,000 Scoville units, "a habañero can measure 500,000 Scoville units—100 times hotter than a jalapeño!" says DeWitt.

Chile connoisseurs say the habañero's fire is short-lived. But when your mouth is on fire, a minute or two can seem like an eternity, so try this pepper at your own risk.

Red-Hot Chile Tips

When it comes to using chile peppers, you're limited only by your imagination (and your courage). Here are a few common—and un-common—uses for these fiery delicacies.

• Spice up a salad with a small amount of chile peppers, suggests DeWitt. If you're using dried chiles, be aware that they tend to be hotter than fresh peppers.

• Mix a tiny bit of chopped chile peppers into mayonnaise or salad dressing, suggests dietitian Nancy Gerlach, R.D., food editor of *Chili*

Pepper Magazine. Or add cayenne or any type of ground chile pepper to barbecue sauce. "But bear in mind that capsaicin is soluble in oil," she notes. Translation: The longer chile peppers sit in mayonnaise or salad dressing, says Gerlach, the hotter these condiments will get. So skimp on the amount of chile you use, at least at first.

•Add chile peppers to your homemade chili. "Both the type and amount of chile peppers you use are matters of personal preference," says DeWitt. "Some people use a base of green chile peppers; others prefer red." Let your taste buds be your guide, he adds.

•Add fresh or powdered chile peppers to your favorite bread recipe, suggests Gerlach, who uses both chopped green chiles and red chili powder in her homemade loaves. "Chiles give bread a real bite," she says.

Mouth Surfing 101

Just as you wouldn't jump into a pool without knowing how to swim, you shouldn't handle—or eat—chile peppers before you know the finer points of going for the burn. These hints can help.

• Chile peppers can burn more than your mouth—they can scorch your skin, too. So after you handle chiles, wash your hands with soap and water before you touch your eyes or face. Better yet, wear gloves while chopping chile peppers, especially if you have a cut on your hand or finger. Also, avoid inhaling the peppers' fiery fumes: "The capsaicin can burn your eyes and lips," says Gerlach.

• It's simpler to add chile heat to a dish than to subtract it, says De-Witt. "So add the chile peppers carefully and taste as you go," he cautions. "It's easy to make the food literally too hot to eat."

• If you're unfamiliar with chile peppers, use some commonsense caution. "See how hot the food is before you start wolfing it down," says DeWitt.

If, despite your best efforts, eating a fiery chile pepper dish leaves you screaming for relief, don't gulp water—that will spread the capsaicin throughout your mouth, says DeWitt. Rather, drink a glass of milk or eat a few spoonfuls of yogurt. Milk contains a protein called casein that can help smother capsaicin's flames. Rice, bananas and bread may douse the flames, too.

CHOCOLATE

The New Health Food?

For as long as it's been around to tempt us, chocolate's gotten a bad rap. Too many calories, too addictive, and often, just too darned easy to overindulge in. Now there's sweeter news about chocolate. Research suggests that it not only doesn't raise levels of LDL ("bad" cholesterol), it increases HDL ("good" cholesterol). The flavonoids found in chocolate may act as antioxidants, which are thought to neutralize the artery-clogging plaque that leads to a heart attack.

Researchers at Pennsylvania State University in University Park found that eating moderate amounts of chocolate as part of an overall healthy diet may indeed help your heart. "An ounce of dark chocolate contains ten times more antioxidants than a strawberry," says Penny Kris-Etherton, R.D., Ph.D., professor of nutrition at Penn State. "In addition, my preliminary research shows that a diet containing about an ounce of chocolate a day increases good cholesterol and prevents bad cholesterol from oxidizing, a process that may lead to heart disease."

Here's how you can sensibly enjoy the sweet benefits of chocolate.

• Think of chocolate as a fun, occasional part of a balanced diet. Its new image as a heart helper doesn't mean that you can have it with breakfast, lunch and dinner. It does contain fat, and too much of that leads to higher cholesterol and weight gain.

• Opt for the dark stuff. Dark chocolate is made with more cocoa than milk chocolate, and premium dark chocolate has even more. While that's not a guarantee of higher levels of antioxidants, you will get an edge from lower amounts of saturated fat.

⌒⋇⌒

CHROMIUM

Big Benefits from a Mighty Mineral

Some of the most intriguing research in the nutritional fight against high cholesterol has to do with a trace mineral whose name reminds most people of the shiny stuff on the bumpers of cars: chromium.

Some studies indicate that chromium, which helps control the way your body uses sugar and fat, may boost the body's stores of "good" HDL cholesterol. "When people who follow a normal diet—which tends to be marginally chromium-deficient—consume more chromium, their cholesterol and triglyceride levels benefit," says Richard A. Anderson, Ph.D., lead scientist at the USDA Human Nutrition Research Center in Beltsville, Maryland, and a leading expert on chromium.

What's more, chromium may help people with glucose intolerance avoid developing non-insulin-dependent (type 2) diabetes. Having diabetes increases the risk of developing heart disease. (See "A Strike against Diabetes" on the opposite page.)

The Cholesterol Connection

Researchers at Oklahoma State University in Stillwater had 21 people ages 60 and over take 150 micrograms of chromium every day for three months. Another 21 people took a placebo.

Chromium takers with normal cholesterol exhibited no change in their cholesterol levels. But chromium takers with high cholesterol saw their total cholesterol go down 12 percent and their "bad" LDL cholesterol plummet 14 percent. Just as important, their levels of HDL cholesterol didn't change.

In a second study conducted at Oklahoma State University, researchers had 24 people ages 55 and over take one of three supplements: chromium (210 micrograms), copper or zinc. After two months, the total cholesterol of the folks taking the chromium fell 12 points, from 217 to 205 milligrams/deciliter. When they stopped taking the chromium, their total cholesterol crept up again. Copper and zinc had no effect on cholesterol levels.

In Jerusalem, 76 heart disease patients—about one-third of whom also had type 2 diabetes—consumed either a 250-microgram chromium supplement or a placebo every day for 7 to 16 months. The total cholesterol of the men in the chromium group didn't change. But their HDL cholesterol increased by 21 to 25 percent.

Investigators at the Medical Hospital and Research Centre in Moradabad, India, had 104 patients with type 2 diabetes follow either a chromium-rich diet (129 micrograms of chromium a day) or their usual

---

A STRIKE AGAINST DIABETES

People with diabetes run an increased risk of developing heart disease. For them, chromium may improve glucose tolerance, which is a measure of how well glucose, or sugar, is absorbed into the blood and transported into the cells, according to Richard A. Anderson, Ph.D., lead scientist at the USDA Human Nutrition Research Center in Beltsville, Maryland.

Most people with diabetes have glucose intolerance, a condition in which blood sugar levels are out of control. That's because insulin, a hormone that helps control blood sugar levels, doesn't work properly. Chromium particularly benefits people who already have diabetes by making insulin work more effectively.

In one study, Dr. Anderson, a leading expert on chromium, had 17 people—8 of whom had mild glucose intolerance—eat a chromium-poor diet. After a month, Dr. Anderson divided these people into two groups. While both groups continued on the low-chromium diet, the first group took 200 micrograms of chromium per day. The second group received placebo pills. Five weeks later, the groups were switched, with the first group receiving the placebo pills and vice versa.

The chromium supplements didn't affect blood sugar levels in the glucose-tolerant folks. But the blood sugar levels of the glucose-intolerant people rose nearly 50 percent less when they were taking chromium supplements than when they didn't take these supplements. The upshot? Chromium may reverse glucose intolerance, says Dr. Anderson.

diets, which contained 69 micrograms a day. After two months, the high-chromium group saw their total cholesterol fall 10 percent, their LDL cholesterol decline 12 percent and their HDL cholesterol jump 7 percent. The cholesterol of the low-chromium group didn't change.

Getting Enough Chromium

The Daily Value for chromium is 120 micrograms. The average American man consumes 33 micrograms of the mineral a day, and the average woman, 25 micrograms. "We collected data on 32 people over seven consecutive days, and not one of them averaged even 50 micrograms of chromium over that one-week period," says Dr. Anderson.

Turkey ham, grape juice, broccoli, unpeeled apples, green beans and whole wheat products are good sources of chromium. So, apparently, are some breakfast cereals. "Total breakfast cereal is very high in chromium," says Dr. Anderson. "One serving contains nearly 27 micrograms of chromium, which is probably as much as you'll get from everything else you eat all day."

But you need to watch the rest of your diet, too, says Dr. Anderson—especially if you have a sweet tooth. Consuming too many highly processed, sugary foods can rob the body of chromium (which is excreted through the urine). According to Dr. Anderson, "Eating lots of simple sugars may also increase your need for chromium supplements because you're consuming fewer chromium-rich foods. So you need to pay attention to your overall diet as well as to the amount of chromium you're getting."

Dr. Anderson recommends taking a multivitamin/mineral supplement containing 50 to 200 micrograms of chromium. "One leading brand contains 100 micrograms of chromium," he says. "That extra 100 micrograms a day can serve as an insurance policy should there be a deficiency in your diet."

If you have diabetes, you may need even more chromium, says Dr. Anderson—about 400 to 600 micrograms a day. Is consuming this amount of chromium safe? Yes, says Dr. Anderson. "We've been studying chromium for decades, and we've never documented a single case of a negative effect," he says. Still, check with your doctor before taking more than a 200-microgram supplement per day.

❧

COFFEE CONTROL

Enjoy Your Java in Moderation

Whether you linger over designer lattes at trendy coffee bars or savor fresh, strong joe from your trusty old percolator, one thing's for sure: When it comes to the relationship between coffee consumption and elevated blood cholesterol, there's controversy brewing.

Some studies suggest that coffee can raise cholesterol levels; others conclude just the opposite. Most of the studies conducted in the United States have found that people who don't drink coffee have higher rates of coronary heart disease than coffee drinkers! In fact, the prestigious Framingham Heart Study concluded that drinking up to five cups of coffee a day may actually have lowered the risk of coronary heart disease, says William P. Castelli, M.D., medical director of the Framingham Cardiovascular Institute, a wellness program at Metro West Medical Center in Massachusetts.

The good news is, consuming moderate amounts of coffee does not appear to raise the risk of heart disease. What's more, some experts say that a cup or two of coffee a day shouldn't significantly affect your cholesterol level. (No large studies have been conducted on the effect of other caffeinated foods or drinks—such as chocolate or cola—on blood cholesterol levels.)

But caffeine can affect the body in other ways. Consumed in large amounts, it can sap bone strength and accelerate the heart rate. Further complicating the coffee/cholesterol issue: the role of nicotine. Some studies note that avid coffee drinkers tend to smoke more than people who drink coffee in moderate amounts, and smoking has definitely been implicated in the development of coronary heart disease.

The Caffeine/Cholesterol Connection

Investigators have conducted numerous studies on the relationship between coffee, elevated cholesterol and heart disease. Results have been inconclusive, however. Some of these studies show that when it comes to coffee and cholesterol, much depends on how the coffee is prepared, according to Dr. Castelli. "Boiled coffee, like the kind drunk in Scandinavia and Turkey, tends to raise cholesterol and the risk of heart disease," says Dr. Castelli. "But filtered coffee does not raise cholesterol or increase the risk of heart disease."

Researchers at Boston University polled 858 women hospitalized with a first heart attack and an equal number of healthy women on their health habits, including coffee consumption. Researchers found that compared with non–coffee drinkers, women who said they drank five to six cups of coffee a day had a 40 percent greater risk of having a heart attack; women who drank seven to nine cups, a 70 percent greater risk. But women who drank less than five cups of coffee a day had no higher risk than women who didn't drink coffee at all.

Investigators at Kaiser Permanente Medical Center in Oakland, California, evaluated the relationship between coffee and tea intake and mortality rate—including deaths from coronary heart disease—in nearly 129,000 people. After an eight-year follow-up period, neither coffee nor tea was found to have increased the overall death rate in these people. Drinking four or more cups of coffee a day was tied to a slightly higher risk of death from heart attack, however.

Researchers at Johns Hopkins Medical Institutions in Baltimore had 100 healthy men drink varying amounts of filtered coffee: 24 ounces of regular coffee, 12 ounces of regular coffee, 24 ounces of decaffeinated coffee or no coffee at all. After eight weeks, the men who drank the 24 ounces of regular coffee a day experienced small increases in their total cholesterol, due to slight rises in their "bad" LDL and "good" HDL cholesterol. The researchers concluded that these small increases in LDL and HDL together "should not affect coronary heart disease risk." That's because small changes in HDL can protect against much larger changes in LDL, explains Dr. Castelli.

In Israel, researchers analyzed coffee and tea consumption and cholesterol levels in 5,369 people. The investigators' conclusion: People who drank five or more cups of coffee a day had higher levels of total cholesterol—as much as 18 milligrams/deciliter higher—than those who abstained from coffee. The researchers also noted that the people who drank the most coffee in their study were also the most likely to have negative health habits, especially smoking. "It is conceivable that the increased cholesterol levels in smokers may be confounded by coffee drinking," wrote the researchers.

Some coffee drinkers may make other lifestyle choices that may be responsible for elevating their cholesterol levels, suggests Connie Diekman, R.D., a dietitian in St. Louis and a spokesperson for the American Dietetic Association. For example, "caffeine tends to stimulate hunger in certain people," says Diekman. "Some people may respond by eating foods that increase their cholesterol levels. But it's difficult to isolate the effect of caffeine on cholesterol and to determine whether the increases in cholesterol are caused by caffeine or by something else."

Watch the Lattes

Most people don't have to be overly anxious about their caffeine intakes, says Robert J. Nicolosi, Ph.D., director of the Cardiovascular Research Center at the University of Lowell in Massachusetts. "In my

---

WHAT ABOUT DECAF?

You drink decaffeinated coffee, so it can't possibly affect your cholesterol. Right? Not so fast. In one study, decaffeinated coffee raised levels of "bad" LDL cholesterol, while regular, caffeinated coffee did not.

Scientists at the Lipid Research Clinic at Stanford University had 181 healthy middle-age men drink several cups of regular, drip-filtered coffee a day. After two months, some of the men switched to decaf; others continued to drink regular coffee. After another two months, the decaf drinkers saw their LDL cholesterol increase significantly. The regular-coffee drinkers experienced no such changes in LDL. Further, the LDL cholesterol levels of the decaf drinkers were 6 percent higher than that of the regular-coffee drinkers.

The researchers' conclusion: It is not the caffeine in coffee but some other factor in the decaf that's responsible for the increase in LDL cholesterol.

But William P. Castelli, M.D., medical director of the Framingham Cardiovascular Institute, a wellness program at Metro West Medical Center in Massachusetts, remains skeptical. "This is just one study," he says.

Heart-Healthy ♡
Indulgences

CHICORY: A COFFEE SUBSTITUTE
THAT CLOBBERS CHOLESTEROL

In the United States, coffee is still the beverage of choice for most people. In countries like The Netherlands and Belgium, however, chicory is used as a wake-up brew, and it seems that they're onto a good thing. Research suggests that chicory is good for the heart.

One study found that chicory reduced cholesterol levels and raised the ratio of HDL to LDL in the blood of the animals tested. Evidence also shows that two substances in chicory, inulin and oligofructose, help the intestinal system by promoting the growth of good bacteria (similar to those in yogurt) and may aid in preventing osteoporosis. Early tests on animals also indicated some good results in preventing and inhibiting colon and breast cancer.

Not sure you're willing to give up coffee? To reap the benefits of chicory, try the following tips.

Try New Orleans–style coffee. You can use chicory to enhance the flavor of your regular java, a popular practice in New Orleans.

Get used to it. Although chicory is slightly bitter, you'll become accustomed to it after a while.

---

view, avoiding caffeine is not one of the lifestyle interventions you need to be most concerned about," says Dr. Nicolosi. While it's possible that caffeine may contribute to elevated cholesterol, he says, "the evidence is very weak at this point."

Diekman concurs. "If you enjoy coffee in moderation and it's not affecting your body—such as accelerating your heart·rate—continue to drink it," she says. "But keep in mind that coffee provides no nutritional value. So make sure it's not crowding nourishing beverages (such as juice or fat-free milk) out of your diet."

Also, pay attention to flavored and specialty coffees, including those served at the local coffee bar, says Barbie Casselman, a nutrition consultant in Toronto. Some coffee beverages contain large amounts of high-fat milk and syrup, so you may be sipping more fat and calories than you realize.

"Most people think that a cappuccino is 6 ounces of coffee and 2 ounces of whipped milk," says Casselman. "But a regular-size cappuccino is actually 2 ounces of espresso plus a cup of milk; in a large cappuccino, there are 12 ounces of milk. If whole milk is used, you might be consuming about 200 calories and eight grams of fat in that 12 ounces of milk. You could eat a dessert for that!"

Coffee Caveats

The jury is out on whether there's an association between coffee consumption and elevated blood cholesterol. But there's less doubt, say experts, that caffeine can affect your nerves—and your bones.

"I consider caffeine to be a mind-altering drug, in the same category as nicotine and alcohol," says Dr. Nicolosi. "Some people are super-sensitive to caffeine and become hyperactive when drinking coffee." These people should consider limiting their consumption of caffeine, he says.

Caffeine may also encourage the development of osteoporosis, the bone-thinning disease that affects many women (and men) later in life, says Isadore Rosenfeld, M.D., author of *Doctor, What Should I Eat?* "Caffeine steals calcium from the body by causing more of it to be excreted in the urine," says Dr. Rosenfeld. He notes, though, that "there's some research to show that drinking a glass of fat-free milk a day can offset the losses caused by coffee. So make sure you're getting plenty of calcium from milk and other sources."

Two health conditions in which some experts advise reducing or completely eliminating caffeine are heart disease and pregnancy. They recommend that people at high risk for heart attack consider drinking less coffee—under four cups a day, according to some research. And while it's not certain whether caffeine can harm a developing fetus, cautious mothers-to-be may choose to avoid caffeine during their entire pregnancies, recommends Evelyn Tribole, R.D., a dietitian in Beverly Hills, California, and author of *Healthy Homestyle Cooking*.

See also Smoking Cessation, Tea

∾❀৯

COOKING

From the Frying Pan into the Steamer

Is there life after fettuccine Alfredo and fried chicken? The answer is a resounding yes. But as more and more health-conscious folks have learned, eating for (rather than to) your heart's content means changing not only what you eat but how you prepare it.

Some of the following culinary tricks help trim the fat from old favorites; other tips update traditional cooking methods with healthier ones. You'll also discover how to sneak low-fat ingredients into your favorite dishes, with your taste buds none the wiser.

As you try new ways of preparing old favorites, you might think of yourself as a culinary explorer, navigating the dangers of the high-fat, high-cholesterol jungle to discover the brave new world of heart-smart cuisine. "The challenge is to cut the fat from our diets while still enjoying our foods," says dietitian Marilyn Guthrie, R.D., manager of health promotion at Virginia Mason Medical Center in Seattle. Once you've met that challenge, you'll get a free bonus: the satisfaction of knowing that you're helping to protect your heart and the hearts of those you care about. So get cooking!

Slimmed-Down Homestyle Favorites

We asked several well-known dietitians and cookbook authors for their advice in creating healthy versions of some high-fat, high-calorie "forbidden" foods. Here are their tasty tips.

Chili and Chowder

Chili con carne. If you choose to add ground beef or turkey to your chili, "stir-fry the meat and drain off the fat before adding it to the pot," says Wahida Karmally, R.D., director of nutrition at the Irving Center for Clinical Research at Columbia-Presbyterian Medical Center in New York City and a member of the American Heart Association's

---

LOW-CHOLESTEROL COOKING 101

Here are the basics of low-cholesterol cookery.

- Trim all visible fat from meat before cooking, advises Nancy Baggett, author of *100% Pleasure: The Low-Fat Cookbook for People Who Love to Eat*. Also, before you eat poultry, you should remove the skin.
- Bake, broil, braise, grill, boil or steam foods, advises dietitian Marilyn Guthrie, R.D., manager of health promotion at Virginia Mason Medical Center in Seattle.
- In baked goods use skim milk rather than whole milk, advises Baggett. "Your taste buds will never notice the difference," she says.
- When stir-frying or sautéing foods, use nonstick cooking spray. Or you can replace each tablespoon of oil in a recipe with a teaspoon of oil plus a few tablespoons of chicken or beef broth, says Baggett.

---

nutrition committee. A better idea: Replace some or all of the beef with beans, which contain virtually no fat and lots of cholesterol-busting soluble fiber, says Karmally.

Clam chowder. Substitute 1 percent milk for whole milk and fat-free evaporated milk for cream, suggests Evelyn Tribole, R.D., a dietitian in Beverly Hills, California, and author of *Healthy Homestyle Cooking*. And if you usually add bacon to your chowder recipe, "use a dash of liquid smoke instead," she says.

Casseroles and Pasta Dishes

Beef stroganoff. Instead of using canned cream of mushroom soup, the traditional ingredient in this family favorite, "mix an envelope of onion-mushroom soup mix with a cup of fat-free evaporated milk and some cornstarch," says Tribole. Bring the sauce to a boil, add the beef and serve over noodles with a dollop of fat-free yogurt, if desired.

Lasagna. "Layer the noodles with vegetables instead of with fatty meats such as sausage," suggests Julia Della Croce, author of *The Vegetarian Table*. She suggests roasting or grilling (not frying) zucchini or eggplant, then layering the vegetables with the noodles. To further defat lasagna, opt for reduced-fat ricotta cheese and light spaghetti sauce.

Spaghetti and meatballs. Substitute a tangy blend of chopped fresh tomatoes, basil, garlic and balsamic vinegar for the traditional meat- or sausage-filled sauce, suggests Dean Ornish, M.D., president and director of the Preventive Medicine Research Institute in Sausalito, California, and author of *Dr. Dean Ornish's Program for Reversing Heart Disease.* For meatballs, "try adding crumbled soy burgers—they taste just like meat," says Dr. Ornish. Or use one of the many vegetable burgers on the market.

Tuna-noodle casserole. Old-style tuna casserole is often prepared with oil-packed tuna, whole milk, fatty cheeses and cream of mushroom soup. As an alternative, JoAnna Lund, author of *The Original Healthy Exchanges*, recommends using water-packed tuna, a cup of reduced-fat Cheddar cheese and a can of Campbell's Healthy Request cream of mushroom soup.

More Main Dishes

Meat loaf. Use egg whites instead of whole eggs, along with very lean ground beef, says Lynn Fischer, author of *Healthy Indulgences.* In fact, consider replacing half of the ground beef with a packaged soy mixture (available in most health food stores), she suggests. To keep the meat loaf moist, add chopped onions, celery, carrots, mushrooms, green peppers or the whites of hard-boiled eggs. Fischer also suggests baking the meat loaf in a perforated pan; suspend the pan over a rack so that the fat can drain off.

Pizza. Lund uses reduced-fat mozzarella, reduced-calorie tomato sauce and "skinny" toppings such as lean ground turkey and fresh vegetables. "I use $3/4$ cup of cheese and about eight ounces of ground meat for a pizza that serves six," she says. "You'll never miss all of that high-fat sausage and cheese."

Quiche. Try making Lund's crustless Cheddar cheese–carrot quiche. She replaces whole milk with nonfat dry milk, eggs with egg substitute and whole-fat Cheddar cheese with three ounces of the reduced-fat variety.

Sloppy joes. Use 90 percent lean ground beef or ground turkey instead of regular ground beef, suggests Lund. To pump up the flavor of this very lean meat, "mix $1/2$ cup of chunky salsa with a can of tomato sauce," says Lund. "I also add a tablespoon of brown sugar substitute, which gives the meat just a hint of Southwest barbecue."

Sauces and Stuffings

Fettuccine sauce. Blend fat-free cream cheese, fat-free milk and fat-free cottage cheese in a food processor for about four minutes, then heat, suggests Fischer. Add ¼ cup of very lean diced ham and 1 cup of peas, if desired, she says.

Quick and healthy gravy. To prepare a tasty make-ahead sauce for chicken, freeze chicken stock in ice cube trays, suggests Sue Chapman, executive chef at the Skylonda Fitness Retreat in Woodside, California. "When you're ready to make the sauce, melt a few cubes, then add a bit of red wine and some fresh herbs such as rosemary," she says. "This sauce delivers the flavor of a traditional gravy without the fat."

Stuffing. Here is Tribole's reduced-fat version of a holiday favorite: Preheat the oven to 350°. Sauté chopped onions, celery and

---

LOW-FAT ALTERNATIVES TO HIGH-FAT INGREDIENTS

Want to make your next meal a cholesterol-busting bonanza? Cut the fat—and the cholesterol—with these heart-smart substitutes.

WHEN YOU NEED . . .	USE . . .
Butter, lard or shortening	Nonstick cooking spray; olive or canola oil
Cream	Fat-free evaporated milk; fat-free milk; 1% milk
Oil or margarine	Applesauce (for muffins and quick breads)
Sour cream	Fat-free or low-fat plain yogurt; pureed 1% cottage cheese with a little lemon juice
Whipped cream	Whipped fat-free evaporated milk
Whole eggs	Egg substitute; egg whites
Whole milk	Fat-free evaporated milk; fat-free milk; 1% milk; reconstituted nonfat dry milk

mushrooms in a nonstick skillet coated with a nonstick cooking spray. Place unseasoned cornbread stuffing in a two-quart casserole, add the sautéed vegetables and some defatted chicken broth, then bake for 30 to 40 minutes.

Miscellaneous Goodies

French toast. Dunk your bread in egg substitute instead of whole eggs, suggests Fischer, and "fry" it in a nonstick skillet coated with a nonstick cooking spray rather than butter. You can enjoy French toast with a small amount of maple syrup, says Fischer; "just don't top it with a big hunk of butter," she advises.

Potato salad. Replace whole hard-boiled eggs with just the egg whites and whole-fat mayonnaise with the reduced-fat or fat-free variety, suggests Fischer. "The fat-free mayonnaise products available today are wonderful," she says. To boost the flavor of this salad, "try adding chopped Spanish onions, celery, dill pickles and scallions," she says.

See also Chicken, Eggs, Fat-Free Milk, Fish, Lean Meat, Margarine, Mediterranean Diet, Vegetables

❧

DESSERTS

Sweet Satisfaction—Guaranteed

If you are watching your cholesterol but can't seem to tame your sweet tooth, don't despair: You can have your cake and eat it, too, while keeping your cholesterol at a heart-healthy level. Low-fat, low-calorie dessert classics such as fresh fruit and sugar-free gelatin can go a long way toward satisfying an urge for something sweet. And if you're hit with an out-and-out craving for chocolate, you can either trim the fat from your favorite home-baked desserts or head to any supermarket: Most now carry a wide array of reduced-fat cookies, cholesterol-free baked goods and fat-free yogurt.

But beware: Some fat-free and cholesterol-free sweets can be loaded with calories. Moreover, indulging in these treats can too often help pile on the pounds—definitely not a heart-smart move. So you'll need to look beyond the "no cholesterol" hype that often adorns these products' labels. On the other hand, treating yourself to an occasional hot fudge sundae most likely won't jeopardize an otherwise low-fat diet, say experts.

Living *La Dolce Vita*

What's for dessert? Try one of these delicious suggestions.

• You can't pick a healthier dessert than fresh fruit. For an extra-special treat, create an elegant fruit salad using exotic fruits such as fresh pineapple, kiwifruit, mangoes and blueberries.

• Put a peeled banana in a plastic bag and pop it in the freezer, suggests Michael Klaper, M.D., health director of the Royal Atlantic Health Spa in Pompano Beach, Florida, and author of *Vegan Nutrition: Pure and Simple.* "When the banana is frozen, slice it and sprinkle it with chopped nuts," says Dr. Klaper. Try freezing seedless grapes, too.

• Jazz up sugar-free gelatin with sliced fresh fruit or a dollop of low-fat whipped topping. Or prepare sugar-free chocolate or vanilla pudding with 1 percent low-fat milk.

• If it's cookies you crave, try one of the many reduced-fat or fat-free varieties on the market. But beware: Low-fat cookies aren't necessarily low in calories—or fat, for that matter. Case in point: Reduced-fat Oreos get 33 percent of their calories from fat, while regular Oreos get 39 percent of their calories from fat. Beware, too, of "cholesterol-free" cookies, cakes and pastries: Many of these products are made with palm or coconut oil—both of which are full of artery-clogging saturated fat—or partially hydrogenated vegetable oil, which contains cholesterol-raising trans fatty acids.

• Screaming for ice cream? Opt for a cup of sherbet, which contains just 4 grams of fat (compared with 24 grams of fat for premium ice cream), or fat-free sorbet. "Ice milk and low-fat or fat-free frozen yogurt are other good alternatives," recommends Lisa Lauri, R.D., nutrition consultant at North Shore University Hospital in Manhasset, New York. Many people enjoy sugar-free fudge bars and fruit pops, too.

• Angel food cake, made with cholesterol-free egg whites, is a luscious low-fat dessert. "Top your piece of cake with sliced strawberries," suggests James W. Anderson, M.D., professor of medicine and

Heart-Healthy ♡
Indulgences

BENECOL BARS: A CHOLESTEROL-LOWERING AFTER-DINNER TREAT

If you enjoy a little treat after a meal, you're in luck: Benecol brand snack bars can wallop cholesterol at the same time they're wowing your taste buds.

Studies show that three servings of Benecol a day lower total blood cholesterol by an average of 10 percent and reduce LDL cholesterol by 14 percent. The cholesterol-clobbering ingredients are plant sterols, which work by blocking absorption of cholesterol by your body. The bars come in chocolate, strawberry and peanut flavors.

Before you start gobbling Benecol bars, though, there are a few things to consider.

Eat them with meals, not in between. This is because the plant sterols have to be in your gastrointestinal tract at the same time as the cholesterol that they block.

Have the bars in place of, not in addition to, dessert. That way, they can work to fight the cholesterol from your main course.

Limit yourself to three a day. Each bar has 130 to 140 calories, so overindulging could translate to weight gain—not a heart-healthy result.

Since Benecol bars do not block saturated fat, a proven enemy of heart health, you can't go crazy with cheese, prime rib and butter just because you're eating Benecol bars. To fully benefit from this heart-healthy indulgence, stick with a diet low in saturated fat.

Despite its cholesterol-reducing ability, Benecol has not been classified as a drug. It's a food with a dietary ingredient—the plant stanol esters—that's been proven to reduce cholesterol levels. (You can use this product as part of a cholesterol-managing diet even if you're taking cholesterol-lowering medication, but it's always a good idea to check with your doctor whenever you consider making significant dietary changes.)

clinical nutrition at the University of Kentucky School of Medicine in Lexington and author of *Dr. Anderson's High-Fiber Fitness Plan*. Or treat yourself to a few tablespoons of whipped topping—it'll cost you just two grams of fat, says Dr. Anderson.

• To lighten up strawberry shortcake, "make the biscuits with canola oil instead of butter and use half of a biscuit per serving rather than a whole one," suggests Susan Purdy, author of *Have Your Cake and Eat It, Too: 200 Luscious, Low-Fat Cakes, Pies, Cookies, Puddings and Other Desserts You Thought You Could Never Eat Again*. Also, try replacing whipped cream with fat-free vanilla frozen yogurt.

• Yearning for a slice of pie? Whip up a treat that is equally tasty but has a fraction of the fat. "Make a low-fat piecrust out of phyllo dough," suggests Marilyn Cerino, R.D., nutrition consultant at the Benjamin Franklin Center for Health of Pennsylvania Hospital in Philadelphia. "Then fill the shell with mounds of strawberries just before you're ready to serve it. It tastes wonderful."

• Substitute low-fat cream cheese for the regular variety in your favorite cheesecake recipe, says Purdy. Or use fat-free cottage cheese: "It's a wonderful addition to cheesecake because it provides a creamy mouthfeel." Put the cottage cheese through a strainer, then puree it in a food processor or blender until it has the consistency of sour cream.

Purdy also suggests reducing the number of eggs you use. If your recipe calls for three whole eggs, "try using one whole egg plus two whites," she says.

• The next time you bake brownies, replace the standard semisweet chocolate with unsweetened cocoa and the butter with a cup of pureed prunes, suggests Purdy. "The prunes keep the brownies moist, and the overall fat content is about one-fifth of the fat in a traditional brownie recipe," she says. Also, "butter" the brownie pan with a nonstick cooking spray.

• You can slim down chocolate cake by replacing a significant portion of unsweetened or semisweet chocolate with cocoa, using fewer egg yolks and reducing the amount of fat, says Purdy. "If the recipe calls for a cup of butter or shortening, for example, use ⅔ cup," she says. To further reduce the amount of fat, substitute fat-free or low-fat yogurt for a small portion of the butter or shortening, says Purdy.

• Defat other home-baked treats. "When you bake a cake, for example, substitute two egg whites for every whole egg," suggests Lauri.

"And if your recipe calls for ⅓ cup of oil, use ⅓ cup of applesauce instead." These substitutions work for boxed mixes, too, notes Lauri.

• To trim the fat from a boxed brownie mix that calls for eggs and oil, "use egg substitute instead of whole eggs and fat-free yogurt in place of the oil," says Janet Lepke, R.D., a dietitian in Santa Monica, California, and a spokesperson for the American Dietetic Association. "The brownies will be chewy and gooey—just as they should be."

When Temptation Strikes

You may never feel cheated by opting for a spicy baked apple over apple pie or fat-free frozen yogurt over premium ice cream. On the other hand, never say never, says Cerino. "If you adore hot fudge sundaes, indulge once in a while," she says. "It's no big deal, as long as you don't have one on a regular basis."

"If you're dreaming of apple pie, have some," adds Sheah Rarback, R.D., director of nutrition at the Mailman Center at the University of Miami School of Medicine. Eat a smaller piece of pie than you would have in the past, suggests Rarback, or spend your fat calories on the pie and curb your fat intake for the rest of the day. "But avoid feelings of deprivation," advises Rarback. "Any food can fit into a low-fat diet. What counts is how often you eat it, how much of it you eat and what else you're eating."

EGGS

Not a Problem for Everyone

Can't remember the last time you ate a three-egg omelette? You're not alone. Many people have cut down on eggs—or even given them up entirely—as part of their efforts to lower their cholesterol.

We consume eggs in many forms, some obvious, such as omelettes, and some not so obvious. Many packaged foods and bottled sauces and dressings contain eggs, and of course, they're used in recipes such as cakes, pastries, pasta dishes and meat loaf.

But you don't have to eliminate eggs entirely. You're probably already cooking delicious dishes using egg whites or commercial egg substitutes (which are a lot tastier than they used to be). You can even eat whole eggs in moderation. Any way you crack it, though, you can savor the flavor of eggs and be kind to your coronary arteries.

Eggs Aren't All Bad

Eggs definitely have their good points. One large egg is brimming with vitamins E and B_{12}, folate, riboflavin, phosphorus and iron and has less than two grams of saturated fat. They pack plenty of protein, too. "Eggs are the best-quality, least expensive protein we can eat," says Wanda Howell, R.D., Ph.D., assistant professor of nutritional sciences at the University of Arizona in Tucson.

So why can't we enjoy eggs as often as we wish? Because "most of the protein in the egg is in the white; all of the cholesterol is in the yolk," explains Dean Ornish, M.D., president and director of the Preventive Medicine Research Institute in Sausalito, California, and author of *Dr. Dean Ornish's Program for Reversing Heart Disease.* The yolk of one average egg contains 213 milligrams of dietary cholesterol—more than two-thirds of the daily limit of 300 milligrams recommended by the American Heart Association (AHA).

The AHA says that healthy adults can eat up to four whole eggs per week but advises people with elevated cholesterol to limit themselves to one whole egg a week. "Because eggs—or more specifically, egg yolks—are a concentrated source of dietary cholesterol, you shouldn't overdo them," says Chicago dietitian Alicia Moag-Stahlberg, R.D., a spokesperson for the American Dietetic Association.

In one study, 25 people were asked to eat 12 eggs a week for six weeks. In 23 of the participants, cholesterol levels stayed the same. In the other 2, LDL cholesterol rose by 25 percent. That translates into a 50 percent increase in the estimated risk of a heart attack.

The term *responders* was used by the researchers to describe the people whose LDL increased. There's no way to know if you'll be a responder, so study author Nancy Lewis, R.D., Ph.D., a nutritionist at

---

LOVE TO BAKE? LOSE THE YOLKS!

You don't have to forgo baking—or eating—your favorite cakes, cookies and muffins because you're cutting back on eggs. Here's how to bake yolk-free treats.

Baking with egg whites. Not using egg yolks won't significantly affect the texture of baked goods, says Evelyn Tribole, R.D., a dietitian in Beverly Hills, California, and author of *Healthy Homestyle Cooking.* "Most likely, you won't notice the difference," she says. She recommends substituting two beaten egg whites for each whole egg.

If you're baking a product that calls for three or four whole eggs, however, substituting that many egg whites may create too much liquid. In that case, you may want to use an egg substitute.

Baking with egg substitute. Some experts suggest replacing each whole egg with ¼ cup of egg substitute, but you can use more or less of this product to suit your taste.

---

the University of Nebraska in Lincoln, recommends that you have your cholesterol checked a month or so after adding eggs to your diet. If your numbers have spiked upward, switch back to egg substitutes. (If you have diabetes, you should avoid eggs completely, according to a Harvard study.)

Evidently, eating eggs doesn't necessarily raise blood levels of cholesterol in everyone. In some cases, people who eat eggs even seem to have lower cholesterol than those who do not. Data from the National Health and Nutritional Examination Survey, conducted by the Centers for Disease Control and Prevention, showed that, after adjusting for age, gender and ethnic background and accounting for lifestyle variables (smoking and physical activity), people who reported eating four or more eggs a week had significantly lower blood cholesterol concentrations than those who reported eating one or fewer eggs a week. The report noted that eggs provide important nutrients and that eating eggs frequently was not associated with increased blood cholesterol levels.

Don't get hung up on eggs and disregard the rest of your diet, though. While cutting back on dietary cholesterol can often help lower your blood cholesterol, "reducing your intake of total and saturated fat will help even more," says Dr. Howell.

Breaking Free of the Yolk

As mentioned, only egg yolks contain dietary cholesterol, which means you can eat as many egg whites as you wish. Doesn't sound like much of a treat, you say? Get creative! Here are some ideas to get you started.

- It's possible for you to create an appetizing breakfast without using whole eggs. "You don't have to sacrifice flavor," says Evelyn Tribole, R.D., a dietitian in Beverly Hills, California, and author of *Healthy Homestyle Cooking.* "Try making French toast with egg whites and fat-free milk. Or make egg-white omelettes stuffed with bell peppers, mushrooms and onions. Chopped green chile peppers work well, too." But don't sauté all of those vegetables in butter. Use a nonstick cooking spray instead.
- Make cholesterol-free *huevos rancheros*, suggests Marvin Moser, M.D., clinical professor of medicine at Yale University School of Medicine and author of *Week by Week to a Strong Heart.* Simply fold scrambled egg whites into a taco or tortilla, then top the eggs with spicy salsa.
- Add chopped egg whites from hard-boiled eggs to tuna salad. Making the salad with reduced-fat or fat-free mayonnaise will slash your intake of dietary cholesterol even more.

Try This Tasty Impostor

Yearning for a plate of steaming scrambled eggs? You can indulge your craving with egg substitutes. These products consist primarily of egg whites, with other ingredients—including fat-free milk, food coloring, vegetable oil and vitamins—added to mimic the taste and texture of real eggs and to boost nutritional value. Most egg substitutes contain zero cholesterol and one to four grams of fat per serving.

Use egg substitute as you would egg whites or even whole eggs. You can make a tasty omelette by adding chopped onions, mushrooms, peppers and reduced-fat or fat-free cheese to egg substitute, for example. Or you can mix this product with flavored bread crumbs to batter-coat baked chicken (without the skin).

If you have tried egg substitute in the past but didn't care for it, you may want to give it another try, says Tribole. "Some of the newer egg

Heart-Healthy ♡
Indulgences

OMEGA-3–ENRICHED EGGS:
FOR MORE HEART-FRIENDLY OMELETTES

You probably never thought you'd see the day when eggs were promoted for their benefits. As unlikely as it seemed, however, that day has arrived.

Scientists have known for some time that omega-3 fatty acids, found primarily in fish, benefit heart health. But omega-3's can now be found in some eggs, since egg producers are feeding hens flaxseed meal, fish meal or marine algae, all of which contain the fatty acids.

The amount of omega-3's that you'll get depends on the product you buy. Choice Eggs, for example, contain 350 milligrams of omega-3 fats per egg.

The omega-3's help you by protecting your heart and improving your mood. Even people with diabetes or high cholesterol can eat up to four eggs a week, and most healthy people can eat up to an egg a day, or seven eggs a week.

Start with this frittata, an "Italian omelette." By combining egg whites and whole eggs, you can reduce fat and cholesterol without compromising taste.

SPINACH AND MUSHROOM FRITTATA

MAKES 4 SERVINGS

½ cup chopped onion
4 ounces mushrooms, sliced
5 ounces frozen chopped spinach, thawed
  and squeezed dry
4 omega-3–enriched eggs

substitutes taste much more like real eggs," she says. And the more brands you try, the more likely it is that you'll find one you like.

There's one advantage of using egg substitute over egg whites, says Tribole: It's yellow, so it looks like the real thing. "If you like scrambled eggs and you're really into eye appeal, use egg substitute," she says. And with more and more restaurants offering omelettes and scrambled eggs made with egg substitute, it's not difficult to follow your program away from home.

6 egg whites
2 teaspoons water
1 tablespoon chopped fresh thyme
1 tablespoon chopped fresh oregano or marjoram
½ teaspoon salt
Pinch of ground black pepper

Coat a large ovenproof nonstick skillet with cooking spray. Warm the skillet over medium heat until hot. Add the onion and mushrooms and cook, stirring frequently, for 4 minutes, or until the mushrooms begin to release their liquid.

Add the spinach and cook, stirring frequently, for 5 minutes, or until most of the liquid has evaporated.

Meanwhile, in a medium bowl, beat together the eggs, egg whites, water, thyme, oregano or marjoram, salt, and pepper. Add to the skillet and swirl to evenly distribute the mixture. Cook over medium heat for 5 minutes, gently lifting the egg mixture from the sides of the skillet with a spatula as it becomes set. Cook until the eggs are set on the bottom but still moist on the top. Remove from the heat.

Wrap the handle of the skillet with 2 layers of heavy foil. Broil 4″ from the heat for 1 minute, or until the top is golden.

Use a spatula to loosen the frittata and slide it onto a serving plate. Cut into wedges and serve.

PER SERVING: 123 CALORIES, 5.2 G FAT (39% OF CALORIES), 13.1 G PROTEIN, 5.7 G CARBOHYDRATES, 213 MG CHOLESTEROL, 0.7 G DIETARY FIBER, 434 MG SODIUM

Three Ways to Have Your Eggs and Eat Them, Too

Sometimes only real eggs will do. If you have elevated cholesterol, most doctors agree that it's smart to stick to the AHA's guidelines and limit yourself to one whole egg per week. Within that guideline, if egg substitute or egg whites just aren't for you, it's possible to occasionally eat whole eggs as part of an overall low-fat, low-cholesterol diet. Try these suggestions.

• "Buy small or medium-size eggs, which contain a little less cholesterol than larger eggs," suggests James W. Anderson, M.D., professor of medicine and clinical nutrition at the University of Kentucky College of Medicine in Lexington and author of *Dr. Anderson's High-Fiber Fitness Plan.*

• Don't scramble or fry eggs in bacon grease or butter, as both are full of saturated fat. Instead, prepare them in a nonstick skillet coated with a nonstick cooking spray. Or try eating eggs hard-boiled or poached, suggests Dr. Howell.

•As mentioned, one egg accounts for most of the AHA's recommended daily intake of dietary cholesterol. "So if you eat an egg on Sunday, make Monday an egg-free or low-cholesterol day," says Sheah Rarback, R.D., director of nutrition at the Mailman Center at the University of Miami School of Medicine. "Concern yourself not with every meal, or even with every mouthful, but with your diet as a whole."

✦

EXERCISE

Work Your Body, Boost Good Cholesterol

If you'd rather surf the Internet than work out at the track or gym, you're not alone. Only about one in ten of us is physically active for a half-hour or more a day. That's unfortunate, because exercise is one of the most powerful weapons we have to keep our hearts healthy and our cholesterol under control.

The good news is, getting into the exercise habit can be easier than you think, even if you haven't worked up a sweat in years. What's more, say many experts, a half-hour of exercise a day is all that it takes to improve your cholesterol profile and reduce your risk of developing heart disease, high blood pressure and diabetes.

Want to exchange a half-hour a day for a lifetime of good health? You can. Read on to find out how.

The Dream Team

According to scientific evidence, exercise helps boost levels of "good" HDL cholesterol, which helps whisk "bad" LDL cholesterol out of the body. "It is thought that exercise's ability to reduce the risk of heart disease comes mostly from its ability to increase HDL cholesterol," says James Rippe, M.D., director of the Center for Clinical and Lifestyle Research at Tufts University School of Medicine in Boston and coauthor of *Dr. James Rippe's Complete Book of Fitness Walking.*

A high HDL level is associated with a decreased risk of heart disease. For every one-point increase in HDL, risk of heart disease sinks by 2 percent for men and 3 percent for women. So if you're a woman who raises your HDL reading from 45 to 55 milligrams/deciliter, you'll slash your risk of heart disease by about 30 percent!

In one study, Japanese researchers looked at the effectiveness of exercise for women with high cholesterol, trying to test the theory that exercise can be helpful in reducing the risk of coronary heart disease even when total cholesterol, low-density lipoprotein cholesterol (LDL) and/or triglycerides, (another type of blood fat implicated in heart disease) don't change.

Twenty-three middle-aged women with high cholesterol participated in 90-minute exercise sessions twice a week for one year and also did home-based exercise three days a week. The women's total cholesterol and LDL did not change significantly after the exercise conditioning, but their triglycerides did decrease significantly (a favorable change in relation to risk of heart disease).

In another study, doctors in Thailand surveyed 3,615 people for their risk factors for heart disease and for how frequently they exercised. The researchers found that people who exercised regularly were more likely to have lower triglyceride levels and resting heart rates. Additionally, levels of beneficial HDL cholesterol were higher in men and women who exercised regularly.

Exercise appears to trigger a chain of physiological events that increase the efficiency of an enzyme called lipoprotein lipase, says Michael Miller, M.D., director of preventive cardiology at the University of Maryland School of Medicine in Baltimore. This enzyme attacks triglycerides. "As lipoprotein lipase breaks down triglyceride-rich particles, it also produces substances that help make HDL," says Dr. Miller. So people who exercise tend to make more HDL and have lower triglyceride levels, he says.

Researchers at the University of Hawaii at Manoa in Honolulu studied the effect of exercise on HDL levels in ten separate studies involving about 700 people. The researchers found that for each 6.2 miles per week that a person jogged, HDL climbed three milligrams/deciliter in both men and women.

Regular exercise can also help you lose weight, which can further improve your cholesterol profile, says William P. Castelli, M.D., medical director of the Framingham Cardiovascular Institute, a wellness program at Metro West Medical Center in Massachusetts. One well-known study determined that for every eight pounds a person sheds, HDL rises about three points. And for every eight pounds gained, HDL declines about two points.

Walk, Cycle, Golf . . . Or Just Scrub the Tub

Think you have to become a marathon runner to raise your HDL and slash your risk of heart disease? Think again. Thirty minutes of moderate-intensity exercise a day can do it, say experts convened by the Centers for Disease Control and Prevention and the American College of Sports Medicine. According to these experts, "the scientific evidence clearly demonstrates that regular, moderate-intensity physical activity provides substantial health benefits."

Experts define moderate exercise as the equivalent of walking two miles at a brisk pace. Other moderate-intensity activities include cycling for pleasure, playing golf (pulling the cart or carrying clubs), cleaning the house, and mowing the lawn with a power mower.

Even better, you can accumulate this 30-minute minimum in short bursts of activity rather than all at once, say experts. So walking instead of driving short distances or pedaling a stationary bicycle while you watch your favorite sitcom can confer substantial health benefits. Best of all, the couch potatoes among us stand to gain the most from increasing their physical activity.

Consult your doctor before you start any exercise program, partic-

---

HOW TO FIND YOUR TARGET HEART RATE

While you work out, periodically check your pulse to be sure you're in your target heart range, suggests James Rippe, M.D., director of the Center for Clinical and Lifestyle Research at Tufts University School of Medicine in Boston and coauthor of *Dr. James Rippe's Complete Book of Fitness Walking.*

To get the low number for your range, subtract your age from 220, then multiply that figure by 0.6. To get the high number for your range, subtract your age from 220, then multiply by 0.85.

If you're 52 years old, for example, you'd subtract 52 from 220, which equals 168. Multiply 168 by 0.6, which equals 100.8 (low number for your range). Multiply 168 by 0.85, which equals 142.8 (high number for your range). Your heart rate should remain between 101 and 142 as you exercise.

Some experts suggest that there's a simpler way to gauge whether you're overextending yourself. "If you can't carry on a conversation during exercise, you're overdoing it," says John McDougall, M.D., creator and head of the McDougall Program at St. Helena Hospital in Santa Rosa, California, and author of *McDougall's Heart Medicine.*

---

ularly if you are a woman over age 50 or a man over age 40, are overweight, have diabetes or heart disease or have ever fainted or experienced chest pains while exercising. And remember to start slowly and listen to your body. "Intense physical activity in people who are not used to it is very dangerous," says Dr. Castelli.

Knock Down Cholesterol with Exercise *and* Diet

While exercise has been proven to lower the risk of coronary heart disease, exercise combined with a low-fat diet can pack an even stronger punch.

Researchers in Germany had one group of men with chest pain exercise at home for a half-hour a day as well as participate in two one-hour group exercise sessions per week. The men also followed a low-fat, low-cholesterol diet. Another group of men was encouraged—but not required—to exercise regularly and consume a low-fat diet.

After a year, the LDL cholesterol of the men who both dieted and

---

CAN PUMPING IRON HELP PUMP UP HDL?

Most health professionals recommend aerobic exercise to help raise "good" HDL cholesterol and protect against heart disease. But there's some preliminary evidence that a nonaerobic activity—weight training—may help lower cholesterol as well.

Researchers at the Department of Veteran Affairs Medical Center and the University of Arizona, both in Tucson, enrolled 46 women in a weight-training program. These women pumped iron for an hour three times a week. Another group of women acted as a control group, sticking to their normal exercise habits.

After five months, the women involved in weight training saw their total cholesterol drop from 184 to 171 milligrams/deciliter. More significantly, however, their LDL cholesterol plummeted by 12 percent, from 116 to 102 milligrams/deciliter, with no significant effect on their HDL levels.

---

exercised dropped an average of 8 percent, and their HDL climbed 3 percent. What's more, only 23 percent of the men experienced progression in existing blockages in their coronary arteries. In another 32 percent, the disease process actually regressed. By contrast, the LDL and HDL cholesterol of the men in the control group didn't change, and 48 percent experienced progression of existing arterial blockages.

Researchers at Stanford University School of Medicine, led by Peter Wood, D.Sc., Ph.D., professor emeritus of medicine, had one group of moderately overweight people follow a low-fat, low-cholesterol diet. A second group followed the same diet but also exercised three times a week. After a year, the exercisers raised their HDL levels by an average of 13 percent. By contrast, the diet-only group raised their HDL 2 percent.

Nine Heart-Healthy Fitness Tips

There's no denying the proven benefits of regular exercise, from a healthier heart to a better shape. So don your sweats and get moving! These tips can help make it easier.

• Put your goals in writing. You're more likely to stick to an exercise program if you know what you want to accomplish and write it down, says exercise physiologist Peter Snell, Ph.D., assistant professor of internal medicine at the University of Texas Southwestern Medical Center at Dallas. "Start keeping a workout log," he suggests. "The log will be a record of what you've accomplished and will help keep you on track."

• Find a workout you enjoy. From fencing to inline skating to yoga, there's a wealth of fitness options that you may not have considered. So explore the alternatives. "When you're having fun being physically active, you're much more likely to keep going, week after week and month after month," says Darlene A. Sedlock, Ph.D., associate professor of kinesiology at Purdue University in West Lafayette, Indiana.

• Go at your own pace. "Don't adhere to the adage 'No pain, no gain,'" says Dr. Sedlock. "Do what you're capable of doing. You'll find that exercise becomes easier and easier."

• Schedule a "happy hour" for exercise. "If you commit to working out at a particular time and place, you'll have a greater chance of meeting your goals," says Dr. Rippe. Try taking an aerobics class during your lunch hour, for example, or enjoy a brisk walk after dinner.

• Work out with a friend who's at a similar fitness level, suggests Dr. Snell.

• Vary your activities—walk on Monday, cycle on Wednesday, play a round of golf on Sunday, and so forth. If you walk regularly, "give yourself a change of scenery by varying your walking route," advises Dr. Rippe. Should you grow weary of your regular Tuesday-night step class, drop in on that Friday-night funk aerobics class that you've been meaning to try.

• If you exercise outdoors, adapt to the weather. "In cold weather, dress in layers that you can remove as your body heats up," says Dr. Rippe. In warm weather, he says, wear loose clothing and drink lots of water before and during your workout. In stormy weather, try walking on an indoor track at the health club or at the mall.

• Add more activity to your day. At work, you might forgo your midmorning coffee break and go on a short walk instead. Or resolve to take the stairs instead of the elevator at least once a day.

• Reward yourself for meeting your exercise goals. Buy a new shade of lipstick or a new tie. Splurge on some new workout gear. "Even a hot bath can be a reward," says Dr. Rippe.

See also Walking

❧

FAT-FREE MILK

Make the Switch

On an airplane flight, Martin Yadrick, R.D., a dietitian in Manhattan Beach, California, and a spokesperson for the American Dietetic Association, asked the flight attendant if he could have some fat-free milk. She said, "No, not unless you order a special meal. But who can drink that stuff anyway? You may as well not drink milk at all!"

If that's the way you feel about fat-free milk, you're not alone. Many an adult, contemplating the switch from whole milk to fat-free, may feel like a kid who has just watched Mom heap broccoli on his plate.

Americans love milk. We dunk cookies in it, use it lavishly in sauces and crave its rich, creamy taste in ice cream, cheese and other dishes. Whole milk is a good source of calcium, which helps prevent osteoporosis, and is rich in protein, minerals and vitamins A and D.

If you're trying to lower your blood cholesterol, however, whole milk doesn't do a body good. One cup of whole milk contains eight grams of fat, 33 milligrams of cholesterol and 150 calories. One study concluded that Americans' passion for whole milk and whole milk products such as cheese "probably contributes substantially to the population burden of coronary heart disease."

But don't assume you have to pass up milk entirely. One cup of fat-free milk contains only 0.4 gram of fat, four milligrams of cholesterol and 85 calories and has all of the nutrients of whole milk, so you won't lose out on the calcium you need to maintain healthy bones.

Best of all, you don't have to give up the taste of coffee with milk, frothy milkshakes and rich, creamy sauces. You can make delicious dishes and desserts with fat-free milk. Read on to find out how.

The Benefits of Moo Juice Lite

A number of studies have compared the effects of whole milk with those of fat-free milk on blood cholesterol. Here's what these studies have found.

Researchers at the University of Minnesota in Minneapolis and other institutions put eight healthy men on a low-fat diet that followed the guidelines of the American Heart Association. For six weeks of a three-month-long study, the men drank two to four cups of whole milk per day. For the other six weeks, they drank an equal amount of fat-free milk. The men's total cholesterol was 7 percent lower, and their "bad" LDL cholesterol was 11 percent lower, on the skim-milk diet than on the whole-milk plan.

These researchers noted that for every 1 percent reduction in total cholesterol, the risk of coronary heart disease drops 2 to 3 percent. Consequently, these experts proposed, healthy men with normal blood cholesterol who drink two to four cups of whole milk a day could slash their risk of coronary heart disease by about 14 percent if they switched from whole milk to fat-free.

Researchers at Kansas State University in Manhattan and Pennsylvania State University in University Park had 64 people supplement their diets with a quart of fat-free milk a day. After two months, people who began the study with total cholesterol of 190 milligrams/deciliter or above saw their total cholesterol decline 6.6 percent and their triglyceride levels drop almost 12 percent. The blood pressure of these men and women dropped as well, perhaps due to the calcium and potassium content of the fat-free milk.

The Skinny on Low-Fat Milk

Using a couple of teaspoons of low-fat milk a day won't hurt you, say experts. But if every day you gulp down a couple of glasses of low-fat milk, which contains either 1 or 2 percent milk fat, you're not trimming as much fat from your diet as you may think.

"Whole milk is 3½ percent milk fat," notes Lisa Lauri, R.D., nutrition consultant at North Shore University Hospital in Manhasset, New York. So if your goal is to lower your blood cholesterol, she says, drinking 2 percent milk isn't the ideal choice.

Keep in mind, too, that water makes up most of the weight of milk. So once water is eliminated from the calculations, 2 percent milk contains 20 percent fat by weight. What's more, 2 percent milk gets 35 percent of its calories from fat, while only 5 percent of the calories in fat-free milk come from fat.

Still not convinced? Here's one more calculation that may help you make the switch to fat-free. If you drink two glasses of 1 percent milk every day for a year, you're swallowing four pounds of fat. Drinking the same amount of fat-free milk, on the other hand, provides less than one-tenth of a pound of fat.

Fake Out Your Taste Buds

These tips can make the transition from whole or low-fat milk to fat-free milk practically painless.

• Drink fat-free milk from a frosted mug. For some reason, lowering the temperature enhances the taste.

• Don't feel you have to switch to fat-free milk right away. "Don't rush it," says Yadrick. "Use 2 percent milk for about a month, then move to 1 percent for the next month. Finally, make the jump to fat-free milk."

• Many people find it difficult to use fat-free milk on breakfast cereals, says Janet Lepke, R.D., a dietitian in Santa Monica, California, and a spokesperson for the American Dietetic Association. "So if you want to use 1 percent milk instead of fat-free on your cereal, it's no big deal," she says. (Consider making the switch to fat-free milk somewhere down the road, though.)

• If you've always used half-and-half or straight cream in your coffee, "try mixing two teaspoons of a liquid nondairy creamer and two teaspoons of 1 percent milk," says Marilyn Cerino, R.D., nutrition consultant at the Benjamin Franklin Center for Health of Pennsylvania Hospital in Philadelphia. "This substitute looks and tastes rich."

• Love bathing your vegetables in a white cream sauce? "Mix a teaspoon each of margarine and flour, then heat for two minutes, slowly whisking in fat-free milk," suggests Cerino. "It makes a delicious sauce."

• If you're yearning for a rich, creamy milkshake, whip up a banana health shake, suggests Evelyn Tribole, R.D., a dietitian in Beverly Hills, California, and author of *Healthy Homestyle Cooking*. Blend one ripe banana, $\frac{1}{4}$ cup of nonfat dry milk, $\frac{1}{2}$ cup of orange juice, one teaspoon of vanilla, a dash of nutmeg and five ice cubes until creamy. "In about a minute, you'll have made a delicious, refreshing drink containing only a trace amount of fat," says Tribole.

༺ঞ৶

FIBER

An Easy Way to Clear Your Arteries

Say "fiber," and many of us think "laxative"—not exactly anyone's favorite noun. But fiber's power to unclog your backed-up plumbing is only part of the story. Numerous studies suggest that fiber can help unplug your arteries, too, by scuttling elevated cholesterol.

Fiber, the part of plant foods that the body can't digest, passes through your system pretty much intact. There are two basic types, soluble and insoluble. Soluble fibers such as pectin, psyllium and guar gum, found in foods such as oat bran, barley, dried beans, peas and apples, seem to help control the way your body produces and eliminates cholesterol.

"Soluble fiber helps lower serum cholesterol," says Alicia Moag-Stahlberg, R.D., a dietitian in Chicago and a spokesperson for the American Dietetic Association. Insoluble fiber, abundant in whole grain products, fruits, vegetables and cereals, is the stuff that helps keep you regular, speeding food through the system and bulking up your stool. While soluble fiber is the cholesterol buster, filling up on grains, beans, fruits and veggies can benefit more than your blood fats. Scientists believe that eating a fiber-rich diet may help reduce the risk of developing colon cancer, diabetes and other ailments as well as heart disease. All in all, good reasons to munch something that crunches—and that doesn't mean chips.

The Benefits of Bulk

Scientists have conducted numerous studies of fiber's power to stomp cholesterol. In one study, James W. Anderson, M.D., professor of medicine and clinical nutrition at the University of Kentucky College of Medicine in Lexington and author of *Dr. Anderson's High-Fiber Fitness Plan*, and his colleagues divided 146 people with moderately elevated cholesterol into three groups. The first group ate their usual diets. The second group followed a low-fat diet that contained 15 grams (about a half-ounce) of fiber. The third group consumed a low-fat diet packed with 25 grams of fiber.

After a year, the low-fat, high-fiber group's total cholesterol had fallen 13 percent, compared with a 9 percent drop in cholesterol for the low-fat group and a 7 percent decrease in the folks who ate their usual diets. Researchers noted that the fiber boost came from common foods easily added to an ordinary diet—one bowl of cooked oat bran cereal, two small bowls of cooked oatmeal or about five ounces of canned beans a day.

In another study, researchers at Stanford University School of Medicine had 16 people consume 15 grams of soluble fiber (including pectin and psyllium) a day. These folks' total cholesterol fell 8.3 percent, and their "bad" LDL cholesterol dropped 12.4 percent, in just one month. Another Stanford study found that cholesterol declined as soluble fiber consumption increased. People who consumed 5 grams of soluble fiber a day for a month lowered their LDL cholesterol by 5.6 percent, while those who consumed 15 grams of soluble fiber saw their LDL cholesterol plunge 14.9 percent.

There's also evidence that adding soluble fiber to a diet already low in fat can further slam cholesterol. Researchers from the United States, Canada and Switzerland had 43 people with high cholesterol follow either a low-fat, high-soluble-fiber diet or a low-fat, high-insoluble-fiber diet for four months. Then the group that had followed the soluble-fiber plan consumed the diet high in insoluble fiber, and vice versa, for another four months. The study participants' total and LDL cholesterol were 5 percent lower when they consumed the diet rich in soluble fiber than when they followed the plan high in insoluble fiber, researchers found.

Researchers at St. Michael's Hospital in Toronto decided to investigate whether a combination of two plant components, vegetable protein and soluble fiber, further reduce cholesterol levels when consumed as part of a diet low in saturated fat. They also looked at changes in apolipoprotein B (apoB), a newly discovered predictor of heart health. Thirty-one men and women with high cholesterol ate two different low-fat, low-cholesterol diets for one month at a time. One diet had a higher amount of vegetable protein (including soy) and twice as much soluble fiber as the control diet.

BEST FOOD SOURCES OF FIBER

Want to clamp down on high cholesterol? Chomp into these foods— they're high in soluble fiber, the kind that helps lower blood cholesterol. Many also supply insoluble fiber, which offers other health benefits.

FOOD	TOTAL FIBER (G.)	SOLUBLE FIBER (G.)
All-Bran cereal (⅓ cup)	8.6	1.4
Apple, with skin (1 small)	2.8	1
Barley, raw (2 Tbsp)	3	0.9
Blackberries (¾ cup)	3.7	1.1
Blueberries (¾ cup)	1.4	0.3
Brussels sprouts (1 cup)	5	2.6
Carrot, raw (1)	2.3	1.1
Chickpeas (½ cup)	4.3	1.3
Corn bran, raw (2 Tbsp)	7.7	0.1
Figs, dried (3)	4.6	2.2
Grapefruit, pink (1)	1.4	0.3
Kidney beans, cooked (½ cup)	6.9	2.8
Lentils, boiled (½ cup)	5.2	0.6
Lima beans, canned (½ cup)	4.3	1.1
Oat bran, dry (⅓ cup)	4	2
Okra (1 cup)	7.3	2.9
Orange (1 small)	2.9	1.8
Pear (1 small)	2.9	1.1
Peas, frozen, cooked (½ cup)	4.3	1.3
Pinto beans, cooked (½ cup)	5.9	1.9
Plums, red, with skin (2 medium)	2.4	1.1
Potato, baked (1)	5	1.2
Pumpernickel bread (1 slice)	2.7	1.2
Raisins, seedless (½ cup)	1.6	0.8
Spaghetti, whole wheat, cooked (1 cup)	5.4	1.2
Spinach, boiled (½ cup)	1.6	0.5
Sweet potato, baked (1)	2.7	1.2
Turnips, cooked (½ cup)	4.8	1.7
Wheat germ, toasted (¼ cup)	5.2	0.8
White/navy beans, cooked (½ cup)	6.5	2.2

Compared with people who ate the low-fat control diet, those who ate the test diet decreased their total cholesterol by an average of 6.2 percent, LDL cholesterol by an average of 6.7 percent, and apoB by about 8 percent. Ratios of LDL to HDL cholesterol, on average, improved by 6.3 percent. The researchers concluded that combining vegetable protein and soluble fiber significantly improved the cholesterol-lowering effect of a low-saturated-fat diet.

Are You Getting Your Fair Share of Fiber?

Many of us consume less fiber than we should, notes Moag-Stahlberg. "Americans consume about 12 grams of fiber (less than a half-ounce) a day," she says. "We should be eating about 25 to 30 grams (about an ounce) per day." Fortunately, it's easy to fiber up your diet. The following tips can help.

• Be sure to eat the skins of fruits and vegetables (such as apples and potatoes) as well as fruits with edible seeds, such as figs and blueberries.

The Coronary Artery Risk Development in Young Adults (CARDIA) Study, a multicenter study that examined heart disease risk factors in young men and women over a period of ten years, showed that young adults who ate at least 21 grams of fiber a day gained eight pounds less than people who ate the same number of calories but less than 12 grams of fiber. Since weight control also helps control cholesterol, that doubles the benefits of fiber.

• Try to get your fiber from foods rather than from fiber supplements, recommends Moag-Stahlberg. Researchers at the N. W. Lipid Research Clinic in Seattle evaluated the cholesterol-lowering effects of a dietary supplement of water-soluble fibers (guar gum and pectin) and mostly non-water-soluble fibers (soy fiber, pea fiber, and corn bran) in people with mild to moderate high cholesterol. They were randomly assigned to receive 20 grams of the fiber supplement or a placebo (inactive substance) daily for 15 weeks. After that period, all of the participants received the fiber supplement for an additional 36 weeks.

Decreases in LDL cholesterol levels, total cholesterol levels, and LDL to HDL ratio were greater in the fiber group. Researchers say that the fiber supplement provided significant and sustained reductions in

LDL without reducing HDL and had the added bonus of not increasing triglycerides (another blood fat) over the treatment period.

However, relying on supplements as your sole source of fiber isn't ideal. The supplements lack other nutrients found in fiber-rich foods, says Moag-Stahlberg. "Fruits and vegetables contain antioxidant vitamins, for example, which may help prevent heart disease and cancer."

• Don't consume a day's worth of fiber in one sitting, advises Susan Kleiner, R.D., Ph.D., a nutritionist in Seattle and author of *The High-Performance Cookbook*. "Eat high-fiber foods throughout the day," she advises. "Don't depend on a high-fiber cereal whose manufacturer claims that you can get all of your fiber in one bowl."

• Drink eight to ten glasses of water a day, advises William P. Castelli, M.D., medical director of the Framingham Cardiovascular Institute, a wellness program at Metro West Medical Center in Massachusetts. Fiber absorbs fluid as it passes through the body, and not drinking enough water can lead to constipation.

• To minimize gas and bloating—common side effects of consuming more fiber—add fiber-rich foods to your diet slowly, says Dr. Anderson.

• Don't gobble fiber to compensate for eating high-fat foods, says Dr. Castelli.

As Dean Ornish, M.D., president and director of the Preventive Medicine Research Institute in Sausalito, California, says in *Dr. Dean Ornish's Program for Reversing Heart Disease*, "A bowl of (oatmeal) is an ideal breakfast, but it won't undo the effects of a ham-and-cheese omelette on the side."

See also Beans, Fruit, High-Fiber Cereals, Oats, Vegetables, Vegetarian Diet

༄❦ఞ

FISH

"Brain Food" That's Good for Your Heart

If you sometimes feel like you're swimming upstream in the fight to lower your blood cholesterol, fish can help you turn the tide. Not only is fish low in saturated fat, but it also contains oils called omega-3 fatty acids, highly polyunsaturated fats that can work small miracles in your body. In most studies, the anchorlike omega-3's have dragged down high cholesterol concentrations to healthier levels.

"Omega-3's appear to decrease blood levels of VLDL (very low density lipoprotein), which is manufactured by the liver," says Peter O. Kwiterovich, Jr., M.D., professor of medicine and director of the Lipid Research and Atherosclerosis Unit at Johns Hopkins University School of Medicine in Baltimore and author of *The Johns Hopkins Complete Guide for Preventing and Reversing Heart Disease.* As VLDL measurements plummet, so may blood cholesterol levels and triglycerides, another blood fat implicated in heart disease. The two most common omega-3 fatty acids are eicosapentaenoic acid and docosahexaenoic acid.

Omega-3 fatty acids also appear to help lower blood pressure, a significant risk factor for heart attack and stroke. Moreover, omega-3's help keep blood platelets from clinging to one another, which can defend against blood clots that may trigger a heart attack or stroke.

Generally speaking, the fattier the fish, the more omega-3 fatty acids it contains, says Margo Denke, M.D., associate professor of medicine in the Center for Human Nutrition at the University of Texas Southwestern Medical Center at Dallas. Interestingly, fish don't manufacture omega-3's. They derive these fats from ocean foods such as saltwater algae and other cold-water vegetation. "So cold-water trout, salmon and mackerel are good sources of omega-3's, while farm-raised catfish isn't," says Dr. Denke. Other fish rich in omega-3 fatty acids include herring and bluefin tuna.

But fish has even more going for it than the cholesterol-clobbering

---

BEST CHOICES FOR OMEGA-3'S

Here's the omega-3 fatty acid content of common varieties of fish. The higher the better, when you're trolling for unwanted cholesterol.

HIGH LEVELS OF OMEGA-3'S

Albacore tuna	Lake trout
Atlantic herring	Pacific herring
Atlantic mackerel	Pacific mackerel
Atlantic salmon	Pink salmon
Bluefin tuna	Rainbow trout

MEDIUM LEVELS OF OMEGA-3'S

Bluefish	Striped bass
Channel catfish	Swordfish
Halibut	Turbot
Red snapper	Yellowfin tuna

LOW LEVELS OF OMEGA-3'S

Atlantic cod	Rockfish
Brook trout	Sole
Carp	Sturgeon
Flounder	Yellow perch
Haddock	Yellowtail
Pacific cod	

omega-3's. Depending on the way it's prepared, fish is also lower in dietary fat than red meat or even poultry. Three ounces of broiled or baked cod, for example, contains 89 calories, 47 grams of cholesterol and less than 1 gram of fat.

Why This School of Fish Gets High Marks

Some of the earliest research into the heart-healthy benefits of fish dates back to studies of the Greenland Eskimos. Researchers found that despite the Eskimos' high-fat diet, they had a low incidence of heart disease, which was linked to their heavy consumption of fish.

Subsequent studies have borne out the connection between omega-3's and heart health. Researchers in Denmark gave 11 men with high levels of blood cholesterol and triglycerides daily supplements of omega-3's in one of three different doses (two, four or nine grams). No matter what the dose, the men's total cholesterol, triglycerides and ratio of total cholesterol to "good" HDL cholesterol declined. Also, the higher the dose of omega-3's, the lower the numbers dropped: Total cholesterol fell 11 percent in the men taking the two-gram dose of omega-3's but dove 22 percent in those taking the nine-gram dose. The men's levels of HDL increased as well, with larger improvements as doses rose.

At Oregon Health Sciences University in Portland, six healthy men alternated between one of two diets that contained varying amounts of total and saturated fat. The men consumed each diet for three weeks, both with and without omega-3 fatty acids.

Researchers found that adding omega-3's to the men's diets significantly reduced their total cholesterol, regardless of how much saturated fat they consumed. Their triglycerides declined even more dramatically—by 41 percent if they were on a high-fat diet with fish oils and 31 percent if they were following a low-fat diet with fish oils.

In South Africa, researchers alternated 28 men and women between a red-meat diet and a fish-only diet that included sardines and salmon. After six weeks on the fish diet, the participants' total cholesterol declined significantly. What's more, their "bad" LDL cholesterol was 9 percent lower on the fish diet than on the red-meat regimen.

Falling for Fish—Hook, Line and Sinker

To reap the maximum benefits from omega-3's, most doctors suggest that we eat fish two or three times a week. But they're less certain of how much fish we should eat. "There's no clear evidence that we need a specific amount of fish oil in our diets," says Dr. Denke. "Fish is a good alternative to chicken and red meat." (But it's best to follow an overall cholesterol-lowering diet that includes plenty of fresh fruits and vegetables, grains and low-fat dairy products as well as fish, meat and poultry.)

The following tips can help you choose and prepare fish that pleases both your taste buds and your ticker.

• Stock up on canned tuna or salmon—it's an easy, inexpensive way to consume omega-3's. To save on calories, buy fish that's packed in water rather than oil.

- If you're buying whole fresh fish, look for clean, tight scales, bright, clear eyes (rather than cloudy or sunken) and red or pink gills. The flesh should also spring back into place when touched.

Further, "fish should have a clean smell, not a strong odor, and the surface of the fish should be moist but not slimy," says A. Garth Rand, Ph.D., professor of food science at the University of Rhode Island in Kingston. Or opt for cleaned, gutted fish—it is more convenient and keeps longer, he adds.

- Unlike red meat, fish has little in the way of visible fat, so in that respect, it doesn't need trimming. But if you're preparing a fatty fish such as mackerel, tuna or swordfish, cut away the darker flesh, says Dr. Rand; it's usually higher in fat.

- The healthiest ways to prepare fish include broiling, baking, grilling and steaming. Don't overcook fish, however. "If the fish's moisture runs out during lengthy cooking, so will some of its nutrients," says Dr. Rand.

You might also stir-fry fish with vegetables, herbs, spices and a small amount of low-sodium soy sauce. "Some kinds of fish make for better stir-fries than others," says Evelyn Tribole, R.D., a dietitian in Beverly Hills, California, and author of *Healthy Homestyle Cooking.* "Stir-fried shrimp, lobster and scallops are wonderful choices."

- If you love fried fish, try this healthy alternative from the American Heart Association: Dip fish fillets in flour and sauté them in a small amount of a polyunsaturated oil. Then place the fish on a heated platter, add some crushed raw garlic and lemon juice to the oil and drizzle the seasoned oil over the fish before serving.

Or "oven-fry" fish, suggests Tribole. "Coat the fish in egg whites—no yolks—and bread crumbs, then bake until crispy," she says. "Squeeze some lemon or orange juice over the fish and sprinkle on some dill."

You might also top the fish with fresh or dried parsley, basil, tarragon or thyme, says Tribole.

- Skewer chunks of fish, onions, tomatoes and peppers and grill fish kabobs. "Preparing kabobs is easy, and most people enjoy them," says Tribole.

- For a quick and healthy meal, microwave fish fillets in a microwave-safe dish along with onions, mushrooms and peppers, suggests James W. Anderson, M.D., professor of medicine and clinical nutrition at the University of Kentucky College of Medicine in Lexington and author of *Dr. Anderson's High-Fiber Fitness Plan.* Or create a quick and tasty entrée by combining fish with your favorite vegetables and grains, says Dr. Anderson.

• If you're dining out, order a seafood appetizer. It will stoke you with omega-3's while it dampens your craving for higher-fat courses. Try boiled shrimp spritzed with lemon juice, smoked salmon served with a platter of raw vegetables, or pickled herring. (For more tips on how to order a heart-smart seafood dinner, see "Best Bets on Seafood Menus" on the opposite page.)

Fish Oil Capsules: A Worthy Alternative?

Can you attack high cholesterol by simply swallowing fish oil supplements?

Maybe, maybe not. A few studies suggest that fish oil supplements, which contain omega-3's extracted from fatty fish, may have some health benefits. One study that examined data on 2,030 men under age 70 who had had heart attacks found that whether the men ate fatty fish (salmon, trout, mackerel or sardines) at least twice a week or took three 500-milligram fish oil capsules a day, their chances of dying during the two-year study period fell 29 percent.

But some doctors say that more studies are needed to prove a relationship between fish oil and lower rates of cardiovascular disease. "There may be instances in which people with very high triglyceride levels can benefit from fish oil capsules," says Wahida Karmally, R.D., director of nutrition at the Irving Center for Clinical Research at Columbia-Presbyterian Medical Center in New York City and a member of the American Heart Association's nutrition committee. "But these capsules have not been shown to lower LDL cholesterol."

Moreover, researchers at Tufts University in Medford, Massachusetts, analyzed popular brands of fish oil supplements and found that they didn't contain sufficient amounts of vitamin E, which is added to help keep the omega-3's in the capsules from breaking down.

So what's the bottom line? "The best way to consume any nutrient is to consume it in food," says Susan Kleiner, R.D., Ph.D., a nutritionist in Seattle and author of *The High-Performance Cookbook.* "Our bodies absorb nutrients most efficiently through food."

BEST BETS ON SEAFOOD MENUS

Craving steamed lobster, broiled scallops or grilled scrod? Go ahead, indulge: According to a national survey, most seafood dishes at mid-priced seafood restaurants are low in fat. It's simply a matter of angling for the right entrées.

The Center for Science in the Public Interest bought take-out portions of a variety of appetizers, side dishes and entrées from 32 seafood restaurants across the country. The center then made a "composite" of each dish (equal portions of nine restaurants' fried fish, for example) and sent it to independent laboratories for nutritional analysis. Among the study's best-bet dishes:

- Clam chowder ($1\frac{1}{2}$ cups, 7 grams of fat)
- Broiled or grilled scallops (six ounces, 3 grams of fat)
- Broiled low-fat fish such as haddock, cod, scrod, sole and flounder (six ounces, 5 grams of fat)
- Blackened catfish (six ounces, 15 grams of fat)

The worst fish dishes: anything fried. That includes fish sandwiches at fast-food restaurants, say experts. "Some people believe that if they order fish sandwiches, they're taking good care of themselves," says Wahida Karmally, R.D., director of nutrition at the Irving Center for Clinical Research at Columbia-Presbyterian Medical Center in New York City and a member of the American Heart Association's nutrition committee. "But eating a fish sandwich may be even worse than eating a plain burger because of all of the fat in the batter."

If you do choose to take omega-3 supplements, however, consult your doctor first, says Dr. Kleiner. Some research shows that large doses of fish oil may thin the blood and may raise the risk of excessive bleeding or stroke. For these reasons, the American Heart Association advises people to take fish oil supplements only under a doctor's supervision.

FLAXSEED

The Artery-Saving Grain

You never know where the next cholesterol fighter is going to come from. A case in point: flaxseed. The fiber and fatty acid in this underutilized grain team up to wield awesome cholesterol-controlling powers.

Flaxseed is brimming with soluble fiber, a substance also found in fresh fruits and vegetables that is known to wallop "bad" LDL cholesterol. What's more, this seed is packed with linolenic acid, a polyunsaturated fat also found in canola oil that's similar to the cholesterol-lowering omega-3 fatty acids in fish. Together, the fiber–linolenic acid offensive may clip double-digit points off your LDL cholesterol.

Much of the credit for discovering flaxseed's ability to lower blood cholesterol belongs to Tom Watkins, Ph.D., laboratory director of the Kenneth L. Jordan Heart Foundation and Research Center in Montclair, New Jersey. Dr. Watkins and his research team have gathered data on flax for years, and his facility has baked enough flaxseed bread to clean out the coronary arteries of a small army.

Dr. Watkins believed that flaxseed's high concentration of linolenic acid might help lower blood cholesterol. To test his theory, he began to bake flaxseed bread, first at home and then in his lab. "The easiest way to consume flaxseed is to bake it into bread," says Dr. Watkins, who experimented with different recipes and formulas. "I ate the bread myself for more than a year, and some of the people in our clinic tried it, too."

In Dr. Watkins's first study, 15 men and women with blood cholesterol above 240 milligrams/deciliter ate three slices of bread made with flaxseed (10 percent of each loaf by weight) per day. The participants also consumed an additional 15 grams of ground flaxseed a day. After three months, these folks' total cholesterol took a tumble from an average of 266 to 248 milligrams/deciliter. And their LDL cholesterol fell from an average of 190 to 171 milligrams/deciliter, a 10 percent decline.

In a second study conducted by Dr. Watkins, 13 people with moderately elevated blood cholesterol ate six slices of either wheat bread or flaxseed bread per day. In this study, flaxseed made up 30 percent of the weight of each loaf. After six weeks of eating the flaxseed bread, the average total cholesterol fell about 10 percent, from 223 to 201 milligrams/deciliter. What's more, LDL cholesterol fell 18 percent, from 162 to 133 milligrams/deciliter—which translates into a probable reduction in heart attack risk of 30 to 40 percent. By contrast, when eating the wheat bread, the participants' total and LDL cholesterol decreased about 6 percent.

FLAXSEED BREAD

MAKES 1 LOAF; 12 SLICES

1½	teaspoons active dry yeast
2	tablespoons + 1¼ cups warm water
3	tablespoons honey
1	tablespoon canola oil
½	teaspoon salt
1	cup flaxseed meal
1¼	cups whole wheat flour
1¾	cups bread flour

In a large bowl, dissolve the yeast in 2 tablespoons of the water. Set aside for about 5 minutes, or until bubbly.

Mix in the honey, oil, salt, and remaining 1¼ cups water. Add the flaxseed meal, whole wheat flour, and 1 cup of the bread flour. Mix well.

Stir in enough of the remaining ¾ cup bread flour to make a soft dough. Turn out the dough onto a lightly floured surface. Knead for 10 minutes, or until smooth and elastic.

Coat a 9″ × 5″ loaf pan with cooking spray. Shape the dough into a loaf and place in the pan. Cover and let rise in a warm place until doubled in bulk, about 1 hour.

Bake at 350° for 40 to 45 minutes, or until the loaf is browned on top and sounds hollow when tapped. Remove from the oven and let cool.

PER SLICE: 179 CALORIES, 4.2 G TOTAL FAT, 0.4 G SATURATED FAT, 4.2 G PROTEIN, 29 G CARBOHYDRATES, 0 MG CHOLESTEROL, 3.0 G DIETARY FIBER, 95 MG SODIUM

Researchers in Canada have studied the effects of flaxseed on blood cholesterol, too. In one experiment at the University of Toronto and St. Michael's Hospital, also in Toronto, nine healthy young women consumed flaxseed flour either in breakfast cereal, soup, juice or yogurt or in bread or muffins. After one month, the flaxseed had reduced the women's total cholesterol by 9 percent and their LDL cholesterol by 18 percent—without lowering their "good" HDL cholesterol.

Bake a Heart-Healthy Loaf

Want to consume flaxseed as part of a low-fat, low-cholesterol diet? Bake a loaf of flaxseed bread, using the recipe on page 97.

You can buy flaxseed in many health food stores that sell grains. Grind the seeds to the consistency of cornmeal using a blender or coffee mill. As a general rule, ⅔ cup of flaxseed yields 1 cup of meal.

Flaxseed bread has a mild, nutlike taste, says Dr. Watkins. While it might go without saying, don't slather flaxseed bread with butter: It's too high in saturated fat. "Some people spread the bread with a little jelly or simply toast the bread and eat it plain," says Dr. Watkins.

Adding flaxseed to your diet may make you feel bloated and gassy, especially at first. To minimize these side effects, eat one slice of flaxseed bread a day and build up to three to six slices a day.

FRUIT

Bananas, Berries and Other Fiber-Full Favorites

When you top your breakfast cereal with strawberries or plunge your fork into a slice of watermelon, it's good news for your taste buds—and your cholesterol level. With few exceptions, fruit is virtually fat-free, so it can help keep your arteries clean as a whistle. Further, fruit is packed with fiber—both the insoluble kind, which helps keep you regular and is associated with a reduced risk of colon cancer, and the soluble kind, proven to whittle down elevated cholesterol levels.

"Grapefruit, apples and strawberries are just some of the good sources of soluble fiber," says Wahida Karmally, R.D., director of nutrition at the Irving Center for Clinical Research at Columbia-Presbyterian Medical Center in New York City and a member of the American Heart Association's nutrition committee. So are pears, prunes and bananas. Most fruits contain a soluble fiber called pectin, a gummy substance that acts as a natural cholesterol cutter.

Prune Your Blood Fats

There's considerable evidence that the soluble fiber in fruits and vegetables helps suck up artery-clogging cholesterol and escort it out of the body.

Researchers at the University of Minnesota in Minneapolis and the University of California, Davis, had 41 men with mildly to moderately high cholesterol add 12 prunes a day to their regular diets. After a month, the men's total cholesterol dropped significantly, from about 230 to 225 milligrams/deciliter, and their "bad" LDL cholesterol fell from 158 to 151 milligrams/deciliter.

In a study conducted in India, researchers had 61 men with high blood pressure—a significant risk factor for heart disease—add between one and two pounds of guava, a tropical fruit, to their regular daily diets. Another group of 59 men consumed their normal diets minus the guava. After 12 weeks, the guava-eaters' total cholesterol had plunged nearly 10 percent, their blood pressure and triglyceride levels had dipped, and their "good" HDL cholesterol had increased 8 percent.

Apparently, the guava-eaters consumed less dietary fat and more potassium—which may help lower blood pressure and protect against stroke—than the guava-free group. But there's nothing special about guava, say experts. The main point is that eating fruit—nearly any kind of fruit—instead of dietary fat can have dramatic results on cholesterol levels.

This conclusion seems to be borne out by another study, also conducted in India. In that study, 621 people at risk for coronary heart disease followed a low-fat, low-cholesterol diet for a month. Next, 310 of the participants were told to increase their intakes of fruits and vegetables to 400 grams (about 14 ounces) or more a day. The folks who maxed out on fruits and veggies saw their cholesterol drop by 6.5 percent, their LDL cholesterol plunge by 7.3 percent and their HDL cholesterol rise by 5.6 percent. Those who didn't eat the extra fruits and vegetables saw no significant improvements.

There's yet another heart-healthy reason to fill up on fruit. Many varieties of fruit—particularly berries, cantaloupe and citrus—are brimming with vitamin C, an antioxidant nutrient that some studies have linked to lower rates of heart disease. Researchers at the University of California, Los Angeles, studied more than 11,000 adults for ten years and found that people who consumed the most vitamin C had a lower risk of dying of heart disease and a lower death rate overall than people with the lowest intakes of vitamin C.

Seven Scrumptious Ways to Feast on Fruit

Sure, you can munch more apples. But there are other ways to meet your fruit quota, too. Try these juicy suggestions.

• Sample the more exotic fruits that you see at the corner fruit stand or in the produce section of your supermarket. Discovering the delights of kiwifruit, passion fruit, mangoes, papayas and fresh pineapple can make eating more fruit an adventure rather than a chore.

• If you're more the classic type, treat yourself to a classic dish: fruit salad. "Slice up some melon, apples, bananas and peaches, and top the fruits with a bit of shredded coconut," suggests Michael Klaper, M.D., health director of the Royal Atlantic Health Spa in Pompano Beach, Florida, and author of *Vegan Nutrition: Pure and Simple*. (Don't overdo the coconut, though—it's very high in saturated fat.) Splash fruit juice over the salad to further boost the flavor, says Dr. Klaper.

• Stir sliced fresh strawberries or bananas into a cup of low-fat or fat-free vanilla yogurt.

• Top pancakes or waffles (prepared with a low-fat mix) with fresh fruit, suggests James W. Anderson, M.D., professor of medicine and

AN APPLE A DAY—AND THEN SOME

The government recommends that we eat five servings of fruits and vegetables a day. While that may sound like a lot, it's really not that hard to do, notes Bettye Nowlin, R.D., a dietitian in Los Angeles and a spokesperson for the American Dietetic Association.

The cup of orange juice and half of a grapefruit that you have at breakfast each count as one serving, says Nowlin. "So does the piece of fruit you have as an afternoon snack," she says. "And when you count the baked potato and cup of salad you might have at dinner—which each count as one serving—five servings isn't that hard to reach."

clinical nutrition at the University of Kentucky College of Medicine in Lexington and author of *Dr. Anderson's High-Fiber Fitness Plan.* Try bananas, strawberries, fresh or frozen peaches, blueberries or even apples sautéed with a pinch of cinnamon and nutmeg. "You can add fruit to pancake and muffin recipes, too," says Dr. Anderson.

• Make a fruit salsa to accompany grilled chicken, fish or turkey. Here's a simple recipe: Peel and dice half of a ripe pineapple, three kiwifruit and half of a melon. Combine with generous amounts of chopped mint and cilantro. Let stand for at least 30 minutes before serving.

• Substitute pureed prunes for butter or margarine in homemade brownies and other chocolate baked goods, suggests Evelyn Tribole, R.D., a Beverly Hills, California, dietitian, in her cookbook *Healthy Homestyle Cooking.* "They add a naturally sweet flavor and chewy texture," she writes. "Best yet, a half-cup of prune puree will save you nearly 800 calories and over 100 grams of fat."

• Whip up a frothy fruit drink. "I call them smoothies," says Dr. Klaper. "Just blend your favorite fruit—say, bananas or strawberries—with some very cold water." These frosty blender drinks are especially refreshing on a summer day, says Klaper.

Fiber Up without Fattening Up

While fruit is a delicious part of a low-fat, low-cholesterol diet, you should keep the following points in mind.

Heart-Healthy ♡
Indulgences

JELL-O WITH FRUIT: COMFORT FOOD FOR CHOLESTEROL

As a child, you probably ate a gelatin dessert when you were feeling sick or just wanted a fun-to-eat treat, especially when Mom added sliced bananas or strawberries.

The best-known brand—Jell-O—has been around since 1897. If you haven't eaten gelatin for years or only make it for your kids, dig out that Jell-O mold. Paired with fruit, gelatin may help control your weight and lower your cholesterol.

Gelatin is a highly purified protein that comes from animal bones and skin. It contains no fat, carbohydrates, or cholesterol. And it's low in calories: only 80 per ½-cup serving. That's good for your heart and your weight. What's more, if you pair your favorite brand of gelatin with diced apples or various citrus fruits, the pectin in the fruits will also help lower cholesterol.

Additionally, studies suggest that gelatin may help people with mild arthritic joint problems. The cartilage in joints, which is damaged by the wear and tear of arthritis, is largely made up of collagen. While trimming fat and collagenous tissue from lean meats and poultry is a healthy practice, it also means that we don't get as much collagen from foods as we used to. Adding gelatin, which is derived from collagen, to your diet may help make up for the shortfall.

First, whole fruits pack significantly more cholesterol-lowering pectin than fruit juices, says Martin Yadrick, R.D., a dietitian in Manhattan Beach, California, and a spokesperson for the American Dietetic Association.

Even a pulp-filled juice can't deliver the fiber of the fruit itself, notes Yadrick. That doesn't mean you shouldn't enjoy your favorite juice; it just means that you should consume whole fruits as well.

Also, don't gorge on avocados. While this fruit is rich in monounsaturated fat, the kind that can help lower LDL cholesterol, you don't want to consume too much of any type of fat.

Happily, you can splurge on an occasional avocado, says Marilyn Cerino, R.D., nutrition consultant at the Benjamin Franklin Center for

Health of Pennsylvania Hospital in Philadelphia. "Many people feel that there's no substitute for really good guacamole," says Cerino. So if a rich, nutty-tasting avocado or spicy guacamole is your weakness, she says, "don't feel like you're cheating—eat it slowly and enjoy it every once in a while."

See also Antioxidants, Apples, Avocados, Pectin

GARLIC

A Pungent Plaque Attacker

If you're fond of garlic-laden pasta (or other dishes prepared with this aromatic member of the onion family), you're automatically paving the way toward good heart health. Numerous studies indicate that garlic may help overpower high cholesterol levels.

Garlic contains allicin, a compound that is activated when the bulb is cut, crushed or cooked. When allicin, which contains sulfur, reacts with oxygen, it breaks down into other compounds that give garlic its distinctive odor and, medical experts speculate, provide its apparent cholesterol-busting abilities.

Garlic also appears to keep blood platelets from clumping together, preventing clots that could trigger a heart attack or stroke. Garlic may also stimulate the blood's natural clot-dissolving processes, which helps get rid of clots that do form.

But this aromatic herb isn't revered for its health benefits alone. Countries from Italy to India have an enduring love affair with the "stinking rose," and Americans consume about 250 million pounds of fresh garlic a year. Should you prefer to help clear your arteries without clearing the room, however, you might opt for garlic supplements, which are odorless pills and powders created to offer the health benefits of garlic without offending the noses of those around you.

Praise the Bulb and Pass the Breath Mints

Garlic hasn't been conclusively proven to reduce cholesterol. But the evidence associating garlic with reductions in total and "bad" LDL cholesterol continues to accumulate.

Researchers at Tulane University School of Medicine in New Orleans gave 42 men and women with elevated cholesterol either 900 milligrams of garlic extract (divided among three capsules) or a placebo every day. After 12 weeks, the total cholesterol of the folks taking the garlic extract fell 6 percent, from 262 to 247 milligrams/deciliter, and their LDL cholesterol plunged 11 percent, from 188 to 168 milligrams/deciliter. (The National Cholesterol Education Program recommends that LDL cholesterol should not exceed 130 milligrams/deciliter.) By contrast, the total and LDL cholesterol of those consuming the placebo fell only 1 and 3 percent, respectively.

In one European study, 40 patients with high cholesterol consumed either 900 milligrams of garlic powder or a placebo every day for 16 weeks. The total cholesterol of the garlic powder group fell an average of 21 percent, and their triglycerides—another blood fat implicated in heart disease—fell 24 percent. The total cholesterol of those taking the placebo declined only 3 percent, while their triglycerides fell 5 percent.

At Tagore Medical College in India, 222 people who had had one heart attack consumed six to ten grams of garlic (about two to three cloves) every day for three or more years. Another group of 210 people took a placebo. Not only did the garlic-eaters' cholesterol levels fall an average of 9 percent, their risk of dying or of having a second heart attack declined as well. The cholesterol of those taking the placebo didn't change.

Experts aren't certain how much garlic might put the kibosh on cholesterol levels. One study that was conducted in the Netherlands concluded that it would take 7 to 28 cloves of garlic a day to help curb cholesterol. Fortunately, a more recent study conducted in the United States indicates that significantly smaller doses of garlic may do some good.

At New York Medical College in Valhalla, Stephen Warshafsky, M.D., and his colleagues in the Section of General Internal Medicine pooled data from five top studies, involving more than 400 people, of garlic's effects on cholesterol levels. According to Dr. Warshafsky's

---

GETTING GARLIC INTO YOUR DIET—GRACEFULLY

Try these handy strategies the next time you eat or cook with garlic.

TO BANISH GARLIC BREATH

Love fresh garlic but hate garlic breath? Try roasting the bulbs, says Audrey Cross, Ph.D., associate clinical professor at Columbia University's Institute of Human Nutrition in New York City. "Roasting garlic helps reduce its odor and some of its sharpness," she says. "Brush the garlic with olive oil to keep it from drying out, then oven-roast the whole clove."

TO AVOID GARLIC-SCENTED HANDS

If you want to use fresh garlic rather than the commercially prepared kind but don't want the smell clinging to your hands, consider investing in an electric chopper, suggests Janet Lepke, R.D., a dietitian in Santa Monica, California, and a spokesperson for the American Dietetic Association. "The garlic is chopped and ready to use in seconds," she says.

---

analysis of the groups studied, one-half to one clove of garlic a day appears to lower blood cholesterol an average of 9 percent.

Tips for Garlic Lovers

Whether you're a card-carrying garlic fan or looking for convenient ways to work this healthful seasoning into your diet, you're sure to benefit from one or more of these tips.

• "One of the easiest ways to use garlic is to chop it up, crush it and sauté it in a little olive or canola oil," says Herbert Pierson, Ph.D., vice-president of Preventive Nutrition Consultants in Woodinville, Wisconsin, and former project director of the Cancer Preventive Designer Food Project at the National Cancer Institute in Rockville, Maryland. "Then you can add it to soups, stews and many other dishes that would benefit from the flavor of garlic."

• Add ground fresh garlic to salad dressings and marinades, suggests Mary Donkersloot, R.D., a dietitian in Beverly Hills, California, a spokesperson for the California Dietetic Association and author of *The Fast Food Diet.*

• If you'd rather not handle fresh garlic, opt for commercially prepared garlic paste or minced garlic in oil. You might also try garlic powder (made from dehydrated and pulverized cloves), garlic oil (distilled from cloves) or aged garlic extract (a water-based garlic product). One large garlic clove is equal to ½ teaspoon of garlic powder and 1 teaspoon of minced garlic.

• Store commercially prepared minced garlic in oil in the refrigerator and garlic powder in a cool, dark cabinet.

• Add garlic to your orange juice. Yes, you read right. "Add an odor-modified substance such as aged garlic extract to orange juice," says Dr. Pierson. "The juice tends to cover up even the slightest garlicky odor." His recipe: Blend three eight-ounce glasses of orange juice, a whole orange and a tablespoon of aged garlic extract liquid.

• If you don't enjoy the taste of garlic, consider trying garlic supplements (available in health food stores and most drugstores). The supplement used in some of the studies Dr. Warshafsky analyzed, Kwai powder tablets, contains the equivalent of 2.7 grams of fresh garlic in each 900-milligram dose. One clove of garlic equals about 3 grams of fresh garlic.

• Don't use garlic salt. This product can be loaded with sodium, which is associated with a rise in blood pressure. What's more, garlic salt doesn't possess the health benefits of fresh garlic.

Consumed in large amounts, garlic can cause a variety of side effects, including heartburn, gas, skin irritation and, rarely, allergic reactions in sensitive people. If you experience garlic-induced discomfort, reduce the amount of garlic you're consuming, advises Dr. Pierson. Or try cooking fresh garlic instead of eating it raw. Cooking garlic tends to weaken its irritating properties, he says.

Also, since garlic has been shown to delay blood-clotting time, consult your doctor before consuming garlic or garlic supplements if you're taking blood-thinning drugs, advises Dr. Pierson.

❦

GRAPE JUICE

The Teetotalers' Toast of Choice

As mentioned elsewhere in this book, drinking wine or other alcoholic beverages in moderation has been shown to boost "good" HDL cholesterol and reduce the risk of coronary heart disease. But if you choose not to imbibe, here's good news: According to one study, grape juice may have the same benefits as wine—including the ability to keep red blood cells from clumping together to form the clots that can lead to a heart attack. While more study is needed, grape juice could be the heart-smart teetotaler's beverage of choice.

The Power of Flavonoids

There's evidence to suggest that antioxidant compounds called flavonoids reduce the "stickiness" of blood-clotting cells called platelets, which in turn lowers the risk of coronary heart disease and heart attack, says John D. Folts, Ph.D., director of the University of Wisconsin Coronary Artery Thrombosis Research and Prevention Lab at the University of Wisconsin Hospital and Clinics in Madison. Flavonoids are found in the skin, stems and seeds of grapes, says Dr. Folts.

In research conducted at the University of Wisconsin, study participants—that is, Dr. Folts and several colleagues—drank varying amounts of grape juice. They then tested one another's blood to monitor its clotting activity. Dogs were also tested, using a different method. The researchers' conclusions: Purple grape juice has the same anticlotting properties of red wine. (Dr. Folts and his colleagues used purple grape juice rather than the red or white variety because darker juice contains more flavonoids, according to Dr. Folts.)

Since there are 800 to 900 different kinds of flavonoids, "it's going to be a massive task to determine which of the flavonoids are the most significant," says Dr. Folts. His research has shown, however, that one of these flavonoids, quercetin, inhibits platelet stickiness—and more. "Quercetin is a better antioxidant than even vitamin E," says Dr. Folts. "So it may also reduce heart disease risk by preventing the oxidation of 'bad' LDL cholesterol." Oxidation is a chemical process that makes LDL cholesterol stickier and thus more likely to cling to arterial walls.

Other research has speculated that resveratrol, a fungus-fighting chemical produced in the skin of grapes, may help lower cholesterol. One study, for example, has shown that purified resveratrol appears to lower cholesterol in rats, and grape juice contains more resveratrol than many wines. But Dr. Folts credits the anticlotting properties of quercetin or other flavonoids with the fruit's potential heart-healthy benefits. "Resveratrol didn't show platelet-inhibiting properties," he says.

How Much Juice?

It appears to take three times as much grape juice by volume to reap red wine's preventive effects, according to Dr. Folts. "Our studies have determined that there's a measurable antiplatelet inhibition from two glasses of red wine," he says. "It would probably take six glasses of grape juice to achieve the same effect."

Besides drinking grape juice, you can boost your intake of flavonoids by eating more fresh fruits and vegetables, suggests Dr. Folts. "There's a fair amount of quercetin in apples," he says. "Broccoli and kale are other good sources."

See also Alcohol, Wine

✦

GUGGUL

A Funny-Sounding Herb with Serious Benefits

Chances are that you've heard about guggul, which has gotten a lot of attention lately because of its heart-healthy benefits.

Guggul is actually the hardened sap, or resin, of an Indian desert tree. This Ayurvedic remedy has been around for many years and has been used by Indian physicians to treat immune system disorders such as rheumatoid arthritis. Now, it's been shown to reduce levels of cholesterol and other blood fats.

How does it work? Some studies, most conducted in India, have identified several active components of guggul. Two of these, gugulipid and guggulsterone, lowered blood fats (cholesterol and triglycerides) significantly in small animals and in people. The theory is that guggul encourages the liver to specifically burn fat and cholesterol.

One study in India showed that 80 percent of people who used guggul extract had a 30 percent drop in levels of cholesterol and other blood fats. Some nutrition experts in the United States remain skeptical about the quality of that research, however.

Although guggul was also a traditional cure for obesity, it's not a magic bullet. It may *help* reduce body fat and cholesterol, but only in tandem with a sensible diet and exercise.

Guggul appears to be quite safe, although some people report occasional stomach upset. People with overactive thyroid should avoid guggul, and it should never be used by pregnant women, because it can stimulate uterine contractions.

If your doctor gives guggul the go-ahead, look for a product marked "standardized" to gugulipids and take 500 milligrams twice a day.

HIGH-FIBER CEREALS

The Perfect Start

Who says cereal is just for breakfast? Certainly not the typical American. In fact, over 90 percent of the folks who responded to one survey said they eat cold cereal at least once a week; 4.5 times per week was the average. Forty percent said they eat cold cereal as a snack. And almost 25 percent said they occasionally break out the cornflakes for dinner!

That's good news—if they're spooning up high-fiber, whole grain products (rather than brands that tend to come with secret decoder rings). Many cereals deliver a day's worth of energy-giving complex carbohydrates, vitamins and minerals in one power-packed bowl and contain little or no fat, says James W. Anderson, M.D., professor of medicine and clinical nutrition at the University of Kentucky College of Medicine in Lexington and author of *Dr. Anderson's High-Fiber Fitness Plan*. Most important, some brands are good sources of cholesterol-clobbering soluble fibers such as oat gum and psyllium, he says. So whether you spoon up a low-fat, high-fiber cereal as an A.M. eye-opener or a P.M. snack, rest assured: You're giving your heart a gift.

Of course, the high-sugar cereals that come in Day-Glo colors and in flavors not found in nature aren't likely to contain much soluble fiber, says Dr. Anderson. Worse, however, are the so-called all-natural cereals that are loaded with nuts, honey, dried fruits and other ingredients that drive their fat and calorie counts sky-high, he says. So to separate the wheat from the . . . er, chaff, prepare to do some sleuthing when you navigate the cereal aisle.

Cholesterol-Slicing Action in Every Spoonful

Several studies have analyzed the effect of high-fiber cereal on blood cholesterol. In one study, researchers at the University of Minnesota in Minneapolis had 58 men with high cholesterol follow a low-fat, low-cholesterol diet for six weeks. For the next six weeks, the men ate the same diet, with one adjustment: They also consumed a pectin-enriched cereal, a psyllium-enriched product or cornflakes, which contained no soluble fiber.

The men's total cholesterol declined about 4 percent on the low-fat diet alone. But the total cholesterol of the men who ate the low-fat diet and the pectin-enriched cereal dropped 6.4 percent, and their "bad" LDL cholesterol fell 8.4 percent. The men who consumed the psyllium-enriched cereal saw their blood fats drop even more: Their total cholesterol dropped 9.2 percent, and their LDL cholesterol plummeted 9.7 percent. The total and LDL cholesterol of the cornflake-eaters didn't change.

In another study, researchers at the University of Toronto had 18 people with high cholesterol eat either a psyllium-enriched cereal or a wheat bran cereal. After two weeks, the total cholesterol of the folks who consumed the psyllium-added cereal dropped 8.4 percent, and their LDL cholesterol plummeted 11.1 percent. The researchers concluded that psyllium-enriched cereal may help cut the risk of coronary heart disease.

Read between the Lines

Stroll down the cereal aisle of almost any supermarket, and you'll see healthful, high-fiber cereals competing for space with box after box of the sugar-coated stuff. Don't be fooled by cereals that look nutritious but aren't. These tips can help you spoon up cereal's maximum cholesterol-busting benefits.

• Choose a cereal that contains at least three grams of fiber and one gram or less of fat per serving, advises Dr. Anderson.

• Consider trying a product enriched with psyllium, which contains a significant amount of soluble fiber, suggests William P. Castelli, M.D., medical director of the Framingham Cardiovascular Institute, a wellness program at Metro West Medical Center in Massachusetts. "Replacing a daily high-fat breakfast, such as eggs and bacon, with a breakfast of cereal high in soluble fiber and fat-free milk can lower cholesterol from 8 to 16 percent within a month," says Dr. Castelli. You'll find several brands on the market, including Bran Buds and FiberWise.

• "Look for as whole a grain of cereal as you can find," advises Michael Klaper, M.D., health director of the Royal Atlantic Health Spa in Pompano Beach, Florida, and author of *Vegan Nutrition: Pure and Simple.* "The box should say 'whole oats,' 'whole barley' or 'whole millet.' One brand to try is Kashi, a blend of oats, long-grain brown rice, rye, barley and other whole grains, suggests Kay Stanfill, R.D., adjunct assistant professor in the Department of Nutritional Sciences at the University of Oklahoma Health Sciences Center in Oklahoma City. "It's a wonderful mix of whole grains, and you can eat it cold or hot," she says.

• Avoid granola-type cereals—they're generally loaded with fat. If you opt for a low-fat granola, however, make sure it's also low in sugar, sodium and calories, says Dr. Anderson.

• To slash fat even more, splash cereal with fat-free milk rather than 2 percent or even 1 percent milk.

• Top high-fiber cereal with fruit. Peaches, strawberries, bananas and raisins will help spike a cereal's fiber content even higher.

• If you enjoy hot cereal but need a break from oatmeal, try barley, roasted buckwheat kernels (also known as kasha) or millet, available in supermarkets and health food stores, suggests Dr. Anderson. These grains are prepared the same way you cook any hot cereal, and they're microwaveable, too. The only catch: Adding cream or butter will negate these cereals' cholesterol-lowering benefits. So stir in your favorite fat-free fruit-flavored yogurt instead, says Dr. Anderson.

• Mix cold cereal with fat-free yogurt for a tasty, low-fat snack.

See also Fiber, Oats, Psyllium

LEAN MEAT

The Red Scare Is Over

If you have elevated cholesterol, you should avoid red meat. Right?

Not necessarily. Despite what you may have heard, experts say that you don't have to forgo steak and burgers entirely to keep tabs on your cholesterol. The key to making red meat part of a low-fat, low-cholesterol diet is to eat smaller portions of leaner cuts, says Susan Kleiner, R.D., Ph.D., a nutritionist in Seattle and author of *The High-Performance Cookbook*.

What's more, red meat is a great source of protein, iron, zinc and B vitamins. But a little bit of red meat goes a long way, and experts still advise against broiling up a steak too often. "Red meat is high in saturated fat, so you shouldn't overdo it," says Janet Lepke, R.D., a dietitian in Santa Monica, California, and a spokesperson for the American Dietetic Association.

Trimming Down the Fat of the Land

For many Americans, eating king-size portions of ribs and roast beef is a thing of the past. According to the USDA, our consumption of beef plummeted from 88.8 pounds per person in 1976 to 62.8 pounds in 1992.

But just when it seemed that Americans would abandon red meat in a mad stampede, the nation's beef producers grew innovative, crossbreeding traditional beef cattle with leaner animals, giving cattle lower-fat feed (which makes their meat less fatty) and sending animals to market at a younger age, when their meat is leaner. Meat packers and butchers are also trimming more visible fat from beef right in the supermarket or butcher shop.

These changes in the raising and packaging of beef mean that in some cases, red meat is lower in fat, cholesterol and calories than it used to be. In fact, the fat content of retail beef declined 27 percent during 1990 and 1991, according to the National Cattleman's Association. Moreover, "some of the leaner cuts of red meat contain less fat than skinless chicken thighs," says Tammy Baker, R.D., a nutritionist in Cave Creek, Arizona, and a spokesperson for the American Dietetic Association.

No Beef with Beef

A few studies have beefed up the argument that red meat can be part of a cholesterol-lowering diet.

In a study at Baylor College of Medicine in Houston, two groups of men with high blood cholesterol levels were placed on a five-week stabilization diet in which 40 percent of their calories came from fat. These men then switched to one of two low-fat test diets in which they ate either chicken breast or lean beef (choice strip loin steak) for five more weeks. The beef contained 8 percent fat, and the chicken, 7 percent fat.

After five weeks, both groups' total cholesterol decreased significantly—7.6 percent for the meat-eaters and 10.2 percent for the poultry-eaters. The men's "bad" LDL cholesterol also dropped significantly on both diets, although not to desirable levels. The researchers concluded that lean beef and chicken are interchangeable in a low-fat, low-cholesterol diet.

In an Australian study, researchers placed ten people on a very low fat diet that contained lean beef with the fat trimmed off. The participants' total cholesterol fell significantly within a week. But when beef fat (in the form of drippings) was added to these folks' diet, their total cholesterol rose. The researchers concluded that it was the beef fat, not the beef itself, that raised blood cholesterol. Further, they wrote, the low-fat diet with lean beef (but without the fat drippings) was just as effective at lowering cholesterol as other low-fat diets that were tested.

A Carnivore's Guide to Cholesterol Busting

To make red meat part of your low-fat, low-cholesterol diet, keep these shopping guidelines and serving suggestions in mind.

• Choose the leanest cuts of meat. If you're shopping for pork, select the tenderloin, leg and shoulder. If you're buying lamb, choose the arm and loin.

• The leanest cuts of beef usually carry the label "USDA select." On average, select beef contains 20 percent less fat than "choice" beef and 40 percent less fat than "prime." Extra-lean ground beef contains just 10 percent fat based on weight.

• You can estimate the fat content of a cut of meat just by looking at it, according to Mary Donkersloot, R.D., a dietitian in Beverly Hills, California, a spokesperson for the California Dietetic Association and author of *The Fast Food Diet*. "Check to see how much white marbling the meat has," she suggests. The more marbling, she says, the more fat.

• Eat red meat only a couple times a week and keep the servings small, advises Baker. "The suggested serving size is about three ounces," she says. "That's a little smaller than the palm of your hand or about the size of a deck of cards." Agrees Dr. Kleiner, "Sixteen-ounce steaks are no longer the way to go."

• Cut away all visible fat from red meat before you cook it. While trimming the fat won't affect its taste much, it will dramatically reduce your intake of fat and calories.

• "If you eat meat, broil it," suggests Gene A. Spiller, D.Sc., Ph.D., director of the Health Research and Studies Center in Los Altos, California, and author of *The Superpyramid Eating Program*. "Let the fat drip off the meat, but don't let it drain on hot charcoal or a hot burner, which will create undesirable fumes."

• If you're wondering how to make do with a three-ounce serving of meat, get creative: Start thinking of meat as an ingredient of the main course rather than as the main course itself, says Evelyn Tribole, R.D., a dietitian in Beverly Hills, California, and author of *Healthy Homestyle Cooking*. "Three ounces of lean ground beef combined with spaghetti is satisfying," says Tribole. "Or stir-fry ground beef and make a low-fat beef stroganoff" using fat-free plain yogurt instead of sour cream.

Lepke agrees that an entrée should most often feature grains and vegetables, with beef playing a supporting role. "Let's say you want to make a stew," she says. "You'd be better off using more chickpeas or vegetables" and less beef.

• Substitute whole or ground turkey or chicken in recipes that call for beef. Make turkey burgers instead of hamburgers, or meat loaf with ground turkey instead of ground beef. "But the less fatty the meat, the drier it can get," says Tribole. She suggests adding a medium-size

Heart-Healthy ♡
Indulgences

CHILI CON CARNE: THE PERFECT WAY TO ENJOY BEEF

Eating the right kind of beef, in moderate amounts, can help lower your cholesterol levels, according to a study conducted at three different American research institutions.

One study looked at 202 men and women with mildly to moderately elevated cholesterol levels. For nine months, five to seven days a week, half of them followed a heart-healthy diet, with lean beef making up 80 percent of the meat they ate. The others ate lean chicken breast for the same period. Both groups lowered their cholesterol—almost 8 percent for the meat eaters and a little over 10 percent for the poultry eaters. The researchers concluded that lean beef and chicken are interchangeable in a low-fat, low-cholesterol diet.

For an inexpensive, convenient, heart-healthy meal, make chili con carne. Combine lean ground beef (sautéed and drained of excess fat), fiber-rich kidney beans and cholesterol-lowering garlic, along with tomatoes, onions and zesty seasonings such as cumin, chili powder and oregano.

THE KINDEST CUTS

The following cuts of beef are among the leanest. Figures are for three ounces cooked. For comparison, the same amount of rib eye steak contains 10 grams of fat and 191 calories, and three ounces of short ribs packs 15.4 grams of fat and 251 calories.

MEAT	FAT (G)	CALORIES
Eye of round	4.2	143
Top roast	4.2	153
Tip round	5.9	157
Top sirloin	6.1	165
Chuck roast	7.6	189
Top loin	8	176
Flank	8.6	176
Tenderloin	8.6	177

grated apple to a pound of ground turkey. "The apple will give the turkey a nice texture without adding extra fat," she says.

• "Marinate meat in something flavorful," suggests Marilyn Cerino, R.D., nutrition consultant at the Benjamin Franklin Center for Health of Pennsylvania Hospital in Philadelphia. A savory marinade: a blend of fresh orange juice, light soy sauce, olive oil, garlic and ginger. "You can use this mixture to marinate strips of meat or chicken that you plan to stir-fry," says Cerino. "And if the meat is tough, marinate it overnight."

• If you're loath to give up burgers and fries, whip up a lower-fat, lower-cholesterol version of this all-American treat. Substitute a whole grain bun for a white-bread bun, and use low-fat or cholesterol-free mayonnaise and low-fat or fat-free cheese instead of regular mayo and American cheese. And put away your deep-fat fryer and opt for spiced, oven-baked home fries instead. Round out the meal with a side dish of baked beans without the salt pork—lots of fiber, virtually no fat.

• If you must have a fast-food burger, order a small burger without fixin's such as cheese, mayonnaise and special sauce, suggests Baker. On the side, opt for a salad with low-fat or fat-free dressing or a baked potato without sour cream or butter.

৵ৡৢ৵

LOW-FAT AND FAT-FREE CHEESES

Slice Away Fat, Not Flavor

If you grew up believing that the four food groups were as sacred as baseball and Mom's apple pie, you may be wondering: How did cheese, once considered an important part of a healthy diet, become so maligned?

If you're trying to lower your blood cholesterol, the answer is all too clear: Eating too much rich, creamy cheese can raise your blood cholesterol and clog your coronary arteries faster than you can say "double-cheese pizza."

But cheer up, cheese-o-philes: "Light" (or "lite") and low-fat cheeses can be just as tasty and versatile as their full-fat counterparts. You might even try fat-free cheeses, which don't contain a speck of fat. And while you may never mistake a low-fat or fat-free cheese for your favorite French Brie, you can make these products a tasty part of a low-fat, low-cholesterol diet. Here's how.

Bypassing Fat City: The Basics

Cheese is little more than a concentrated form of milk. It takes about eight pounds of milk to create a single pound of most cheeses. In many full-fat cheeses, 60 percent or more of their calories come from fat, and one ounce of Cheddar, Swiss, Monterey Jack or Muenster contains eight to ten grams of fat. Just reading a cheese label with those kinds of numbers is enough to make your arteries slam shut!

The good news is that the dairy industry has responded to the public's demands for healthier cheese by introducing some products that get 10 percent or less of their calories from fat and contain two grams or less of fat per ounce. So if you can walk past the Camembert, the Brie and other exotic (and fatty) selections in the deli section of the supermarket and follow a few basic guidelines, you can still say "cheese" with a smile.

The key to choosing heart-healthy cheese, say experts, is to become a dedicated label reader. Select cheeses with low amounts of total fat and saturated fat and low percentages of calories from fat, advises Sheah Rarback, R.D., director of nutrition at the Mailman Center at the University of Miami School of Medicine.

"Choose a cheese in which the percentage of fat is lower than the percentage of protein," says Gene Spiller, D.Sc., Ph.D., director of the Health Research and Studies Center in Los Altos, California, and author of *The Superpyramid Eating Program.* A product that is 20 percent fat and 15 percent protein, for example, should stay out of your shopping cart, says Dr. Spiller.

Also, when it comes to controlling blood cholesterol, a cheese's fat content is more important than its amount of dietary cholesterol, says Ruth Lowenberg, R.D., a dietitian in New York City. The American Heart Association recommends that adults eat less than 300 milligrams of dietary cholesterol per day. Don't be misled, however: A one-ounce serving of American cheese contains 26 milligrams of cholesterol but nine grams of fat—a hefty amount if you're trying to follow a low-fat diet.

A Tip from the French

Just can't give up your favorite full-fat cheese? You might try doing as the French—the world's most prolific cheese eaters—do, says Audrey Cross, Ph.D., associate clinical professor at Columbia University's Institute of Human Nutrition in New York City.

"The French eat very high fat cheeses," says Dr. Cross. "But they eat tiny amounts of them, along with a lot of bread and fruit. Americans tend to eat hunk after hunk of cheeses that aren't as satisfying, trying to attain some satisfaction.

"If we would eat foods that taste good, we'd eat less of them, because we'd be satisfied," continues Dr. Cross. "Try eating an ounce of your favorite cheese instead of five ounces of a variety that you don't enjoy as much. And eat the cheese with bread and a piece of fruit instead of with fatty crackers."

Low-Fat or Fat-Free?

If you're looking to knock a few points off your blood cholesterol by slicing your intake of fatty cheese, you might try low-fat or fat-free cheeses. Here's how these products compare.

Low-fat cheeses. At three grams or less of fat per ounce and about 20 to 50 percent less fat than full-fat cheeses, these products look and taste much like their higher-fat counterparts, says Alicia Moag-Stahlberg, R.D., a dietitian in Chicago and a spokesperson for the American Dietetic Association. Low-fat products even melt like their full-fat counterparts, making them perfect for sauces and toasted cheese sandwiches. "Most people are quite happy with low-fat cheeses," says Moag-Stahlberg. If you're already following a low-fat diet, you may want to select a low-fat cheese over a fat-free product, she says.

Fat-free cheeses. These products contain the barest amount of fat, if any at all. But finding a fat-free cheese that tastes like the real thing can be tricky. Here's why. Whole milk cheese gets its characteristic consistency, texture and flavor from butterfat. To make fat-free cheese, the dairy industry replaces butterfat with fat substitutes, milk solids or other ingredients. "Fat-free products tend to have different textures than low-fat cheeses," says Moag-Stahlberg. "They don't melt as well, either." What's more, fat-free cheeses tend to have very mild flavors—what some people might call bland.

But many people have learned to enjoy fat-free cheese. Their secret? Using a little culinary ingenuity. "If you're using a cheese that has more than 50 percent fat reduction by weight, you may need to find a creative way of preparing it," says Lowenberg, "combining it with other foods to give it more flavor."

Tasty Tips for Cheese Junkies

The kind of cheese you choose—and the way you use it—can make all the difference. These hints can help.

• Look for low-fat "impostors." Chances are there's a low-fat or fat-free alternative for your favorite type of full-fat cheese, including Cheddar (Healthy Choice Fat-Free, Cracker Barrel Light), mozzarella (Kraft Healthy Favorites, Alpine Lace Low Moisture Part-Skim), Swiss (Light 'n' Lively Singles, Kraft Light Naturals) and American (Weight

Heart-Healthy ♡
Indulgences

GORGONZOLA AND CHEDDAR CHEESE:
STRONG FLAVOR, BIG BENEFITS

In small amounts, cheese can be a diet good guy.

A 1½-ounce serving of Cheddar offers about 300 milligrams of calcium, as much as a glass of milk. Cheese also contains a type of fat called conjugated linoleic acid, or CLA, which scientists are investigating as a new weapon against breast cancer. Additionally, eating cheese at the end of meals can protect your teeth against decay.

Still, all this good news comes with a gentle reminder that cheese has a lot of saturated fat. That 1½-ounce serving packs 9 grams of it, and that's not great for your heart. So, while we're not telling you to cut cheese out of your heart-healthy diet altogether, it's best to consume it in small portions. Experts suggest choosing extra-sharp Cheddar or Gorgonzola because their strong flavors will satisfy your taste buds in smaller amounts. Here are some other tips for indulging in real cheese.

Know your Gorgonzola. Be on the lookout for it at the next party you attend, or serve it at your own bash. Gorgonzola has a light ivory surface, and its interior is marbled with blue-green veins. The American Dairy Association says that it tastes great with sweet crackers and walnuts (which are well-known for their cholesterol-cutting power).

Avoid temptation. At home, help yourself to one serving of cheese, then wrap the rest and store it right away.

Watchers Slices, Kraft Free Singles). "Do some taste testing," says Evelyn Tribole, R.D., a dietitian in Beverly Hills, California, and author of *Healthy Homestyle Cooking.* "You may find that there's a considerable difference in taste among brands of the same type of cheese."

• Try combining small amounts of a higher-fat cheese with a low-fat or fat-free product. "You might add cubes of low-fat mozzarella to a salad, then sprinkle the salad with blue cheese," says Lowenberg. "You'll get a wonderful cheesy flavor without using a large amount of the higher-fat cheese."

• Using condiments can give a fat-free cheese some extra zip. "If you're using a fat-free cheese in a sandwich, you may not be able to get away with adding just lettuce and tomato," says Lowenberg. "Try spreading on some horseradish or chutney, which will enhance the cheese's flavor."

• To make a delicious dip, blend 2% cottage cheese with a dry salad-dressing mix, suggests Lowenberg. If a dip recipe calls for sour cream, substitute a mixture of 2% cottage cheese and low-fat yogurt, she says.

• Substitute fat-free cream cheese for the full-fat product in no-bake cheesecakes and refrigerated desserts. Or toss fat-free cream cheese with hot pasta (along with your favorite herbs and spices) for a creamy, Alfredo-type sauce.

• Love the taste of creamy cheeses such as Brie? Try this mock Brie dish, suggests Sue Chapman, executive chef at Skylonda Fitness Retreat in Woodside, California: Mix one part Brie cheese, four parts fat-free cream cheese and some rosemary, shape into rounds and dip in bread crumbs. Then bake.

• The next time you make lasagna, substitute reduced-fat ricotta cheese for the whole milk product. A half-cup of reduced-fat ricotta contains 9.8 grams of fat, compared with 16.1 grams in the same amount of the whole milk stuff.

• As mentioned previously, fat-free cheeses don't melt very well. So don't use these products to top casseroles, advises Tribole. "Fat-free cheese will look like toasted coconut," she says. "I'd use a low-fat cheese instead." Similarly, fat-free mozzarella works better baked into lasagna than on a pizza, she notes. But if you want to use a fat-free cheese in a sauce, "try shredding it very finely," Tribole suggests. "It will melt nicely."

MARGARINE

Take a Second Look

We ate 28 percent less butter in the 1990s than we did in the 1970s. Many men and women who are watching their cholesterol have abandoned butter: About three of every four Americans spread margarine on their morning toast.

Now, however, we're hearing about significant evidence suggesting that trans fatty acids, a type of fat found in margarine as well as a lot of snacks and baked goods, raise "bad" LDL cholesterol, lower "good" HDL cholesterol and increase the risk of heart attack.

Thankfully, the news isn't all bad. Much depends on the type of margarine you select. The more liquid margarine is (such as tub and liquid forms), the fewer trans fatty acids it contains.

The Pumped-Up Fat

Trans fatty acids are by-products of innovations in food technology. Margarine is made mostly from unsaturated oils, such as corn, canola and safflower, to name a few. Unsaturated oils are liquid at room temperature. To solidify them, manufacturers pump them up with hydrogen in a chemical process called hydrogenation. "Hydrogenation makes fats harder," says Sheah Rarback, R.D., director of nutrition at the Mailman Center at the University of Miami School of Medicine. "A stick margarine is more hydrogenated than a soft tub margarine, for example."

Hydrogenation also creates trans fatty acids. Ironically, when unsaturated fatty acids are chemically combined with hydrogen, they become more saturated.

Despite this, however, some experts, including the American Heart Association, still say that it's better to opt for margarine over butter. Why? Because butter has more artery-clogging saturated fat, which has been proven to elevate blood cholesterol and raise the risk of heart disease. Butter contains about seven grams of saturated fat per tablespoon; margarine has only about two grams per tablespoon.

"Studies show that while both trans fatty acids and saturated fat increase LDL cholesterol, saturated fat has a greater effect on cholesterol," says Alicia Moag-Stahlberg, R.D., a dietitian in Chicago and a spokesperson for the American Dietetic Association. Further, we consume far more saturated fat. "About 3 percent of our total calories come from trans fatty acids, compared with 12 to 13 percent from saturated fat," she says.

How Margarine Got a Bad Rap

The margarine controversy began some years ago, when a Dutch study found that trans fatty acids elevate cholesterol levels. Some experts noted that the people in the three-week study consumed about four times more trans fatty acids than the average American. Subsequent studies added fuel to the trans fat fire, suggesting that even smaller amounts of trans fats could help clog coronary arteries.

Perhaps the most persuasive of these investigations was the Nurses' Health Study at Harvard Medical School, which analyzed the health habits of about 87,000 women. The study concluded that women who ate four or more teaspoons (or pats) of margarine a day were 66 percent more likely to develop heart disease than women who consumed less than one teaspoon of margarine a month.

The evidence is mixed, though. International studies show that societies that eat the most butter have higher heart attack rates, says William P. Castelli, M.D., medical director of the Framingham Cardiovascular Institute, a wellness program at Metro West Medical Center in Massachusetts. Also, he says, a highly regarded clinical trial called the Finnish Hospital Study found that people who ate margarine lowered their cholesterol by about 15 percent and cut their heart attack rates roughly in half over a six-year period compared with people who ate butter.

Select the Healthiest Spread

For now, say experts, your best bet is to concentrate on cutting back on saturated fat. If you're still using butter, switching to margarine can be a good start.

"You will dramatically lower your intake of saturated fat and your intake of trans fatty acids, since many margarines have lower levels of trans fatty acids than butter," says Dr. Castelli.

THE FULL SPREAD ON MARGARINE

Regular margarine. Diet margarine. Margarine-butter blends. What sets them all apart? More than you'd think. This guide, with the most healthful options leading the list, can help you sort out the spreads.

Powdered butter. You can sprinkle this nonfat alternative over moist, hot foods such as vegetables and pasta.

Diet margarine. These products, also known as light margarines, contain high amounts of water and weigh in at about half of the fat and calories of regular margarine. Also, they frequently contain fewer trans-fatty acids than butter.

Regular margarine. These products get 100 percent of calories from fat, but the fat is primarily polyunsaturated. Also, most varieties are cholesterol-free.

Vegetable oil spreads. These products typically contain less than 80 percent fat by weight. But according to some experts, they may not be any better than regular margarine.

Margarine-butter blends. These products typically contain from 15 to 40 percent butter, so they are likely to have more saturated fat and cholesterol than regular margarine. "They should be avoided," says William P. Castelli, M.D., medical director of the Framingham Cardio-vascular Institute, a wellness program at Metro West Medical Center in Massachusetts.

With so many varieties of margarine to choose from, picking a truly heart-healthy product can be tricky. These guidelines can help.

• First and foremost, select a margarine that contains no more than two grams of saturated fat per tablespoon, advises the American Heart Association. "Choose only margarines that list water as the first ingredient," advises Dr. Castelli. These products are low in trans fatty acids as well as in saturated fat, he explains. "And avoid margarine that lists partially hydrogenated vegetable oil as the first ingredient," he says. Instead, use products with naturally occurring, unhydrogenated oil such as canola or olive oil when possible. In processed foods, choose those made with unhydrogenated oils over those made with hydro-genated or saturated fat.

• Consider switching to a new cholesterol-lowering spread, such as

Benecol and Take Control, which is made with plant stanol esters (see "Heart-Healthy Indulgences" on page 126). These spreads can be used by people of any age. Finnish researchers investigated the safety and cholesterol-lowering effectiveness of plant stanol ester margarine in 81 healthy six-year-old children already consuming diets low in saturated fat and cholesterol. Their families replaced 20 grams (about four teaspoons) of the children's dietary fat intake with either plant stanol ester margarine or regular margarine for three months. At the end of the study, the group consuming plant stanol ester margarine reduced total and LDL cholesterol concentrations by 5.4 and 7.5 percent, respectively. The serum HDL cholesterol and triglyceride concentrations, among other markers, remained unchanged. Evidently, plant stanol ester margarine lowers total and LDL cholesterol levels without side effects in healthy children who already consume a low-saturated-fat, low-cholesterol diet.

• Avoid stick margarine, as it tends to be highly hydrogenated. Opt for soft, tub-style margarine instead. "The softer the margarine, the lower its content of trans fatty acids and saturated fat," says Alice H. Lichtenstein, D.Sc., assistant professor of nutrition at Tufts University in Medford, Massachusetts, and a scientist at the Jean Mayer USDA Human Nutrition Research Center on Aging in Boston.

• Select a brand with the highest percentage of polyunsaturated fat, advises Dr. Lichtenstein. You might opt for products made from safflower, sunflower, corn or soybean oil.

• If possible, select a liquid or semiliquid spread, particularly for cooking, says Dr. Lichtenstein. When she compared three different diets—a baseline diet with 35 percent of calories from fat, a corn oil margarine–enriched diet with 30 percent of calories from fat and a liquid corn oil–enriched diet with 30 percent of calories from fat—the liquid corn oil was found to cut LDL cholesterol by 17 percent compared with the baseline diet. The corn oil margarine cut LDL by 10 percent compared with the baseline.

• Skip the spread altogether. "We've been raised to think that we should smear something on our toast," says Dr. Lichtenstein. "But if we eat tasty bread, we may not need to." Another option: Top your toast with a small amount of jelly or jam, which contains no saturated fat.

• Avoid products that contain "partially hydrogenated vegetable

Heart-Healthy ♡
Indulgences

BENECOL AND TAKE CONTROL:
GOOD FOR TOAST, SALADS, AND YOUR CHOLESTEROL

There are two new products at the supermarket—Benecol and Take Control spreads and salad dressings—that contain unique substances that help reduce cholesterol. The functional ingredients are plant stanol esters, which block absorption of cholesterol by the body.

A study reported in the *American Journal of Cardiology* showed that when Benecol was used by people taking cholesterol-lowering statin drugs, it reduced LDL cholesterol levels by an additional 17 percent compared with the cholesterol levels of people who took statin drugs and used a placebo spread.

Another study, reported in the *Journal of Nutrition*, showed that plant stanols lower total and LDL cholesterol by blocking cholesterol absorption from the intestine. Because the stanols essentially cannot be absorbed, they are great cholesterol-lowering agents. Plant stanol esters at a level of 2 to 3 grams a day have been shown to lower LDL cholesterol by 10 to 15 percent without side effects.

To get the benefits, three daily servings of Benecol and two of Take Control are recommended. (One serving of spread is $1\frac{1}{2}$ teaspoons; one serving of salad dressing is 2 tablespoons.)

Benecol and Take Control spreads are available in regular and reduced-fat versions. Benecol dressings come in ranch, creamy Italian, Thousand Island and French-style flavors, and Take Control is available in reduced-fat Italian, ranch, and blue cheese. If your cholesterol is high, and you use margarine or salad dressing, these products are good options. (You can use them as part of a cholesterol-managing diet even if you're taking cholesterol-lowering medication, but it's always a good idea to check with your doctor whenever you consider making significant dietary changes.)

oil," another term for trans fatty acids. "In particular, watch out for fried foods, cakes and cookies," says Dr. Lichtenstein.

The bottom line: Experts advise consuming all fats—including margarine—in moderation.

෴

MEAL FREQUENCY

Nibble Away at High Cholesterol

It sounds too good to be true: being able to eat all day long and lower your blood cholesterol in the process. But there's some evidence that "grazing"—eating many small meals or snacks throughout the day rather than the more customary three squares a day—can help shave a few points off your cholesterol level.

But don't confuse eating more often with consuming more calories, say experts. Grazing on hot fudge sundaes and hero sandwiches will benefit neither your cholesterol level nor your shape. "We're recommending not that people eat more calories but that they divide their daily caloric intakes into smaller meals," says Elizabeth Barrett-Connor, M.D., professor and chair of the Department of Family Medicine at the University of California, San Diego.

The good news is that studies indicate that the cholesterol-lowering benefits of eating smaller, more frequent meals seem to take effect without changing your overall diet. How's that for a dream come true?

It Pays to Graze

Grazing may be the natural way to eat, says Dr. Barrett-Connor. "We evolved from people who ate frequent, small meals when they could," she says. "Occasionally, they would get a big kill and gorge. But Americans gorge nearly every night—and that's an unhealthy way to eat."

The body manages smaller meals more efficiently, explains Sharon Edelstein, a research scientist at George Washington University in Washington, D.C. "Humans were meant to be grazers, and that's the way our bodies perform best," she says. "If you pound your body with a lot of food once or twice a day, you may be giving it too much to deal with. If you put food into your body more slowly, you'll process it more efficiently."

Dr. Barrett-Connor agrees. "Eating more meals consisting of less food is more physiologically efficient," she says. "If you throw large amounts of fat and calories at the body all at once, it won't be able to manage them as well. It's more than the body can metabolize." So fueling up only once or twice a day may make it easier for dietary fat to collect in the coronary arteries, leading to elevated cholesterol levels, says Dr. Barrett-Connor.

If you'd like more evidence that eating smaller portions may affect heart health, Marla Mendelson, M.D., assistant professor of medicine at Northwestern University Medical School in Chicago, suggests looking at countries that have lower incidences of cardiovascular disease than the United States, such as Japan and China. "The people in these countries eat smaller portions," says Dr. Mendelson. "This may aid the digestive process, so you're not completely overwhelming the mechanism in the liver with too much food and asking the liver to process it." Overloading the liver may eventually cause free-floating fat and cholesterol to be deposited in the arteries, she says.

Four (or More) Meals Are Better Than One

Researchers found that when laboratory animals ate large, infrequent meals rather than small, frequent ones, their blood cholesterol increased. Multiple feedings resulted in reduced heart disease risk factors—and longer lives, says Dr. Barrett-Connor.

Studies conducted on humans appear to bear out the conclusions of the animal research. Edelstein and Dr. Barrett-Connor, along with other colleagues, studied the diets of more than 2,000 people. They found that the total cholesterol of people who ate four or more meals a day was almost nine points lower than those who reported eating one or two meals a day, says Dr. Barrett-Connor. Also, the frequent eaters' "bad" LDL cholesterol averaged six points lower than that of the infrequent eaters, she says. And while the grazers tended to consume more fat, calories and cholesterol than the two-meal group, their blood cholesterol was still lower, and they were less likely to be obese.

Researchers in New Zealand had 19 healthy men and women with normal blood cholesterol levels consume their usual low-fat diets—with one difference: These folks alternated between eating three meals a day and eating nine meals a day. They spent two weeks on each diet. When the participants followed the nine-meal plan, their total cholesterol fell 6.5 percent, and their LDL cholesterol dropped 8.1 percent. If every 1 percent change in total cholesterol translates to a 2 percent change in the risk of coronary heart disease, wrote the researchers, "then theoretically, there could be a mean 13 percent reduction in the risk of coronary heart disease when meal frequency is increased from three to nine meals a day."

When Canadian researchers had seven men consume 17 small meals or snacks a day, the men's total and LDL cholesterol fell 8.5 percent and 13.5 percent, respectively. The researchers theorized that the smaller meals caused the body to produce less insulin, which in turn decreased levels of a certain enzyme needed by the liver to process cholesterol.

Eat Like a Bird—All Day

Thinking of joining the graze craze? These tips can help.

• People who eat breakfast generally eat more meals a day than people who don't, says Dr. Barrett-Connor. "Breakfast-eaters also are more likely to snack throughout the day than people who diet all day long and eat gigantic dinners," she says. In fact, people who skip breakfast to "save" calories end up spending them—with interest—in the long run. "Their bodies store up fat for the famine they think is coming," says Dr. Barrett-Connor.

• Many weight-control experts recommend that people eat a small snack between meals and another snack before bedtime, says Dr. Barrett-Connor. Snacking between meals provides the body with the same amount of calories but is more physiologically efficient, she says. "Avoid foods high in fat or sugar—they have no nutritional value," advises Dr. Barrett-Connor. "Fruits and vegetables are great choices."

༺❦༻

MEDITERRANEAN DIET

Eat Like Zorba to Heal Your Heart

Pasta redolent with garlic and drizzled with olive oil. Vegetable stew bursting with sun-ripened eggplant and seasoned with herbs. Fresh seafood and hearty bean salad. And hunks of crusty bread to sop up every last drop of sauce or vinaigrette.

Are you salivating yet? Well, go ahead and *mangia*, because eating like this can actually be good for your heart. Just ask the Mediterraneans. The folks in the countries along the Mediterranean Sea—Italy, Greece, southern France and Spain, to be exact—tend to be a

---

THE MEDITERRANEAN DIET PYRAMID

The Harvard School of Public Health, the Oldways Preservational and Exchange Trust and the World Health Organization Regional Office for Europe have endorsed the Mediterranean Diet Pyramid. This dietary model, an alternative to the USDA Food Guide Pyramid, is modeled on the traditional diets of the Mediterranean region around 1960 (before heavy influences from other nations).

The first two levels of the Mediterranean pyramid and the USDA pyramid are similar. Breads, cereals and grains comprise the "base" of each model, while fruits and vegetables comprise the next largest segments.

Then the two plans diverge. The USDA pyramid recommends two to three servings of meat, poultry and fish (along with dried beans, eggs and nuts) per day, while the Mediterranean pyramid recommends that poultry and fish be consumed a few times a week and red meat only a few times a month.

Further, the USDA pyramid recommends that fats and oils be used "sparingly." The Mediterranean pyramid recommends the liberal use of olive oil virtually to the exclusion of all other fats, especially saturated fats such as butter and margarine.

little healthier and live a little longer than people in northern Europe and the United States. Consider these facts.

- According to the World Health Organization, French men and women have a lower than usual incidence of heart attack. So do Italians, especially Italian women.
- In 1990, 243 men and 132 women per 100,000 people in the United States died of heart disease, according to World Health Organization statistics. The same figures for Italy were 139 men and 64 women per 100,000; for Spain, 106 and 47; for Greece, 137 and 59; and for France, 91 and 40. Quite a comparison.
- On average, Greeks live three years longer than Americans (74.3 versus 71.6 years).

What makes the Mediterranean diet so healthy? First, individual components of traditional Mediterranean dishes—garlic, olive oil, grains, beans—have cholesterol-lowering powers of their own. And second, this diet brings together these components in a cuisine now respected for its healthy ways.

Lessons from the Southern Rim

The first to pick up on the Mediterranean mystique was Ancel Keys, Ph.D., of the School of Public Health at the University of Minnesota in Minneapolis, who along with his colleagues launched the Seven Countries Study. Begun in the late 1950s, this benchmark study sought to prove a link between diet and coronary heart disease in almost 13,000 middle-age men throughout the Mediterranean, Northern Europe, Japan and the United States.

After a lengthy follow-up period, Dr. Keys, now professor emeritus of public health at the University of Minnesota, and his team discovered that men from Italy and Greece—especially Greece—died less often from coronary heart disease than men from Finland, northern Europe and the United States.

What Dr. Keys hypothesized decades ago has been embraced by a multitude of eminent medical experts: Diet and heart health are inextricably linked.

But what do Mediterranean people eat—or not eat—that seems to protect their tickers? "The specifics may vary from one Mediterranean country to another, but in general, these populations eat less red meat and more fish," says Barbara Levine, R.D., Ph.D., associate clinical professor of nutrition in medicine at Cornell University Medical College in New York City. Mediterraneans also eat fewer fat-laden dairy products and more fruits, vegetables and grains than Americans. "To eat like Mediterraneans, you'd consume half as much whole milk, cream and butter and 45 percent less red meat," says Dr. Levine. Further, Mediterraneans tend to drink more red wine, which when consumed in moderation can boost levels of HDL, the "good" cholesterol, and limit the risk of heart disease. (See "Salut—In Moderation" on page 134.)

"Mediterranean people are also more physically active than Americans," notes Audrey Cross, Ph.D., associate clinical professor at Columbia University's Institute of Human Nutrition in New York City. "They ride bicycles to work or walk when we might drive, which tends to decrease both their incidence of obesity and their rate of cardiovascular disease."

A Prudent—But Not Spartan—Cuisine

Thus, a number of factors appear to contribute to the Mediterranean people's health and longevity. But perhaps the biggest reason for this region's notable dearth of heart disease, some experts theorize, is its reliance on monounsaturated rather than saturated fat.

The traditional Mediterranean diet averages 35 to 40 percent of total calories from fat. So does the typical American diet. But the American diet is laden with artery-clogging saturated fat, found in animal-derived foods such as red meat, in whole milk dairy products and in processed convenience foods. Mediterranean cuisine, on the other hand, tends to be richer in artery-saving monounsaturated fat, particularly olive oil. In the Mediterranean region, the per capita consumption of olive oil has averaged as high as two to three tablespoons per day. The typical American, on the other hand, consumes about three tablespoons of olive oil every four months. But given the popularity of low-fat cooking and a cholesterol-conscious population, we might use more olive oil in the near future.

In an editorial in the *New England Journal of Medicine*, Walter Willett, M.D., Dr.P.H., professor of epidemiology and nutrition at the Harvard School of Public Health, and his colleague Frank M. Sacks, M.D., associate professor of medicine and nutrition, endorsed the traditional Mediterranean diet, saying that it's just as low in saturated fat and cholesterol as a typical low-fat diet. "The Mediterranean alternative—using monounsaturated fat as a major dietary component—appears to be at least as healthful" as following a low-fat diet, they wrote, and "may be an even better way to improve (blood cholesterol levels)." Further, they wrote, eating the Mediterranean way "will provide more variety and greater satisfaction to many." That's good news for those of us with higher-than-average cholesterol—and hearty appetites.

Eat as in Rome—At Home

If you're used to a diet of beef and butter, the Mediterranean diet may seem a little . . . well, foreign. But many Americans have found that Mediterranean cuisine is as delicious and inexpensive as it is health promoting. Here's how to add the Mediterranean touch to your table.

• Eat less red meat. "In Italy, the focus of the meal is pasta, and meat is more of a side dish," says Wahida Karmally, R.D., director of nutrition at the Irving Center for Clinical Research at Columbia-Presbyterian Medical Center in New York City and a member of the American Heart Association's nutrition committee. "By following the Italian approach and consuming less meat, you can reduce your intake of saturated fat."

• Replace butter and other saturated fats with monounsaturated fat, particularly olive oil. Drizzle this fragrant oil over pasta, steamed vegetables and baked potatoes, for example. Or use it to sauté onions and vegetables. Better yet, use an olive oil cooking spray.

• Eat more fresh vegetables. They're packed with cholesterol-reducing soluble fiber and antioxidant vitamins, which experts speculate may help keep "bad" LDL cholesterol from a damaging chemical reaction called oxidation. (Oxidized LDL becomes stickier and clings to artery walls, experts theorize.) Prepare a French-style ratatouille (an eggplant-based vegetable stew) by simmering onions, eggplant, zucchini and tomatoes with herbs and spices. Serve with crusty French bread, sans butter.

• Consume more whole grains, advises James W. Anderson, M.D., professor of medicine and clinical nutrition at the University of Kentucky College of Medicine in Lexington and author of *Dr. Anderson's*

SALUT—IN MODERATION

In Italy, France and Greece, a bottle of red wine is as much a part of a meal as the robust cuisine and the hearty laughter around the table. But if you don't drink, don't start for the sake of your heart, say experts.

"I advise people to limit their intakes of alcohol to seven drinks a week," says James W. Anderson, M.D., professor of medicine and clinical nutrition at the University of Kentucky College of Medicine in Lexington and author of *Dr. Anderson's High-Fiber Fitness Plan*. (A drink is frequently defined as 4 ounces of wine, 12 ounces of beer or $1\frac{1}{2}$ ounces of liquor.)

Should you opt to enjoy an occasional glass of vino, there's no need to fret about the wine's year or its bouquet—or its color, for that matter. Red and white wine may be equally beneficial for raising "good" HDL cholesterol, according to Tom Watkins, Ph.D., laboratory director of the Kenneth L. Jordan Heart Foundation and Research Center in Montclair, New Jersey. And when it comes to wine's apparent heart-healthy benefits, he continues, an inexpensive California Chablis is just as good as the priciest French Bordeaux.

High-Fiber Fitness Plan. Many varieties, such as barley and oats, are packed with soluble fiber. Try whole wheat pasta rather than the white-flour variety, suggests Dr. Anderson. Or you might try combining seasoned vegetables with bulgur or couscous (which contains more fiber than white rice) to make a spicy Spanish-style pilaf.

• Eat more legumes. Chickpeas, lentils and white beans, mainstays of Mediterranean cuisine, are great sources of low-fat protein and are rich in soluble fiber. Try the classic Italian dish *pasta e fagioli* (pasta with beans) or enjoy a French-style white-bean salad.

• Use more garlic. Besides adding its distinctive flavor and aroma to foods, this aromatic herb may contain certain components that help lower cholesterol. Add minced garlic to pasta dishes, soups and stews, sauces and grilled fish. Or whip up a pot of garlic broth, a popular French staple. Peel and slice six cloves of garlic. Place them in a one-quart saucepan with two cups of water, one bay leaf, one tablespoon of olive oil and some fresh sage. Simmer for 15 minutes, strain into mugs and enjoy.

• Italians like to taste their pasta. So don't overload this inherently healthy dish with fatty sauces or toppings. "Use marinara sauce (a meatless tomato sauce) rather then heavy meat sauces and cheeses," advises Dr. Anderson. Or toss with lightly steamed vegetables—broccoli, zucchini, red peppers—and fresh basil, and add a little Parmesan for pasta primavera.

• Don't overdo the olive oil. "Olive oil is a fat," stresses Tammy Baker, R.D., a nutritionist in Cave Creek, Arizona, and a spokesperson for the American Dietetic Association. "Just because it's a monounsaturated fat doesn't mean you should use a lot of it. Your best bet is to get 30 percent or less of your total calories from fat."

See also Alcohol, Antioxidants, Exercise, Fish, Garlic, Monounsaturated Fat, Olive Oil, Wine

❧

MONOUNSATURATED FAT

The Fat Your Arteries Will Love

Virtually everyone now knows that eating too much fat is hard on the heart as well as on the hips.

As you may have heard, however, one type of fat—monounsaturated fat—isn't so fiendish after all. This fat—found in significant proportions in canola oil, olives and peanuts—generally maintains or even raises heart-saving HDL cholesterol while scuttling "bad" LDL cholesterol. The difference between saturated fat, which contributes to the waxy buildup in arteries, and artery-scrubbing monounsaturated fat is primarily a matter of chemistry. (More about this later.)

Make no mistake: Monounsaturated fat is still fat, and doctors generally advise cutting back on all fat, including the monounsaturated kind. Even so, however, it's nice to know that not all fat is strictly off-limits. Here's what you need to know about mono.

Why Nuts Are Better Than Nachos

Why bake with canola oil rather than butter? Or snack on a handful of nuts rather than the same amount of chips? The answer lies in the chemical makeup of fats.

All fats are made up of carbon, hydrogen and oxygen atoms. Saturated fat is found primarily in red meat, whole milk dairy products and tropical oils (coconut and palm oils). This type of fat is stuffed, or saturated, with the maximum number of hydrogen atoms and is usually solid at room temperature. Unsaturated fat, which includes both monounsaturated fat (abundant in olive and canola oils, along with certain plant foods such as nuts and avocados) and polyunsaturated fat (plentiful in corn, sunflower and safflower oils) contains fewer hydrogen atoms. The less dense unsaturated fats are usually liquid at room temperature.

Most foods contain varying amounts of saturated, polyunsaturated and monounsaturated fats. Most doctors would agree, though, that cholesterol-conscious folks would do well to cut back on foods laden with saturated fat. In fact, some doctors believe that the Mediterranean region's reliance on mono-rich olive oil, coupled with its limited consumption of saturated fat, contributes to the Mediterranean people's unusually healthy hearts and squeaky-clean arteries. Further, several physicians from the Harvard School of Public Health, along with the World Health Organization Regional Office for Europe and the Oldways Preservational and Exchange Trust, have endorsed the traditional Mediterranean way of eating as a healthy alternative to the typical saturated fat–soaked American diet.

These Oils Foil Blood Fats

Study after study points to monounsaturated fat's cholesterol-pounding power. In Spain, researchers put 78 men and women on a diet enriched with sunflower oil. After 12 weeks, the participants switched to an olive oil–based diet. Total cholesterol hadn't budged in the men after an additional four months and had increased 9 percent in the women, who followed the diet for seven months. But there was a significant change: The olive oil plan also increased HDL levels—by 17 percent in the men and 30 percent in the women.

In another study, researchers in Israel put 17 young men on one of two diets. The first group followed a diet rich in monounsaturated fat (olive oil, avocados and almonds). The second group consumed a carbohydrate-based diet. Both diets contained similar levels of saturated and polyunsaturated fats. After three months, the men consuming the mono-rich diet switched to the carbohydrate plan, and vice versa.

After another 90 days, the researchers tested the men's blood cholesterol. The findings? When the men followed the mono-rich diet, their total cholesterol fell by nearly 8 percent, and their LDL levels plunged about 14 percent. No such beneficial changes occurred while the men were following the carbo-based plan.

Heart-Healthy ♡
Indulgences

OLIVES: KEEP YOUR HEART YOUNG

Want to hold off Father Time for a while and lower cholesterol as well? Start enjoying olives, which are tasty treats that can do both.

Olives get a big health bonus from where olive trees grow—the sunny climes of California and the Mediterranean region. Blazing sunshine produces a bounty of anthocyanins, flavonoids and phenols, natural plant substances that fight oxidation caused by the sun's ultraviolet light. Inside your body, these phytochemicals fight the oxidation that may cause aging.

Like the oil they produce, olives are rich in monounsaturated fat, which helps clobber cholesterol and reduce blood clotting, another risk factor for heart disease. As a bonus, monounsaturated oil may also offer some protection against breast cancer.

Eight large black olives or 10 stuffed green olives have a mere 45 calories and 5 grams of fat. But olives do have one potential drawback: They're salty. A serving of 10 large green olives may contain more than 900 milligrams of salt. For people who are sodium sensitive, putting them at risk for high blood pressure, a healthy sodium limit is 2,400 milligrams day. So, if you're a huge fan of olives, try to limit other sources of salt in your diet.

To benefit from olives without overindulging, use them in some of your favorite dishes.

- Scatter them on a pizza with no cheese and extra sauce.
- Serve them alongside vegetables, low-fat dip and zesty cheese.

More recently, two British studies evaluated the cholesterol-lowering effectiveness of a diet high in monounsaturated fatty acids. One studied healthy middle-aged men, and the other studied young men with a family history of coronary heart disease. At the end of both studies, total and LDL cholesterol levels were significantly lower in the men who ate the diet high in monounsaturated fats than in those who had the control diet higher in saturated fat. The researchers concluded that diets in which saturated fat is partially replaced by monounsaturated fats can achieve significant reductions in total and LDL cholesterol concentrations, even when the same amount of total fat and calories are consumed.

A study by researchers at Harvard University and Brigham and Women's Hospital in Boston showed that dieters who ate large amounts of monounsaturated fats lost weight. The primary source of monounsaturated fat in the study was peanut butter.

A Fat by Any Other Name

There's no doubt about it: Replacing the saturated fat in your diet with unsaturated oils can do your heart good. But don't go hog-wild even with monounsaturated oils, experts advise. "Don't pour them over foods," says Michael Klaper, M.D., health director at the Royal Atlantic Health Spa in Pompano Beach, Florida, and author of *Vegan Nutrition: Pure and Simple.* "I generally recommend using a tablespoon or two a day at most."

A small amount of oil can go a long way. You might drizzle a bit of olive oil on a crusty piece of Italian bread for lunch and use the remaining allotment on your salad at dinner. Or lightly coat a skillet with it. "Rather than pouring olive oil in the pan, just brush the bottom with a light coat of oil," suggests Dr. Klaper.

In a nutshell: "Don't increase your intake of monounsaturated fat. Decrease your consumption of saturated fat," advises Evelyn Tribole, R.D., a dietitian in Beverly Hills, California, and author of *Healthy Homestyle Cooking.* "And if you pay attention to food labels, it's so easy to cut back."

See also Canola Oil, Mediterranean Diet, Olive Oil, Polyunsaturated Fat

~❧~

MUSHROOMS

Take a Tip from the Japanese

Stuffed, stir-fried or sautéed, mild or robust, mushrooms are both familiar and mysterious. While you may remember when smooth, creamy white button mushrooms routinely topped a T-bone, you've no doubt noticed more exotic fungi in the produce section of the local grocery store.

But mushrooms may be more than just another food fad or salad fixin'. Long believed by the Japanese to help prevent and treat cancer, mushrooms—namely, the common button mushroom and the rich-tasting shiitake mushroom—may also help lower cholesterol, according to several studies. Research to date on mushrooms' potential cholesterol-cutting powers has been limited but intriguing.

The Magic of Mushrooms

So you wouldn't have guessed that mushrooms might contain cholesterol-cutting powers? That's understandable; after all, these pungent vegetables are about 90 percent water. But the remaining 10 percent contains a mother lode of nutrients, including potassium, calcium, riboflavin, niacin and iron.

What's more, some mushrooms are rich in protein and contain all of the essential amino acids. Essential amino acids, which are necessary for life, can't be manufactured by our bodies; we have to obtain them from food. Mushrooms also contain phytochemicals, or plant substances that may help fight disease, according to Robert Beelman, Ph.D., professor of food science at Pennsylvania State University in University Park.

Since the late 1960s, researchers at the National Institute of Nutrition in Tokyo have conducted tests on the effectiveness of shiitake mushrooms on blood cholesterol. In one study, researchers had young women eat 90 grams of fresh shiitake mushrooms (about five mushrooms) a day. Their average cholesterol level declined 12 percent in a week. When researchers conducted a similar experiment with 30 people over age 60, cholesterol levels fell 9 percent in a week.

In another study, also conducted at the National Institute of Nutrition, researchers had people add 60 grams of butter a day to their diets. These butter-laden diets raised their cholesterol by 14 percent in a week. These folks then consumed 90 grams of shiitake mushrooms a day along with their butter-rich diets. After a week, their average cholesterol level dipped 4 percent.

Fungi Power—Experts' Tasty Tips

While the jury is still out on mushrooms' power to lower cholesterol, these earthy-tasting vegetables can enliven almost any dish, from casseroles to stir-fries. Try these delicious suggestions. *Caution*: Never eat wild mushrooms.

• Select mushrooms with smooth, unblemished caps, because they're the freshest, says Mindy Hermann, R.D., a nutrition consultant in Mount Kisco, New York.

• Toss sautéed mushrooms with white or brown rice. And forgo the butter or margarine: You can sauté three to four cups of mushrooms in a teaspoon of oil in a nonstick skillet on medium heat, says Nancy Baggett, author of *100% Pleasure: The Low-Fat Cookbook for People Who Love to Eat*.

• Add shiitake mushrooms to stews, vegetable dishes or pasta, suggests Faye Levy, author of *Faye Levy's International Vegetable Cookbook*.

• Use sautéed mushrooms as a topping for chicken, says Evelyn Tribole, R.D., a dietitian in Beverly Hills, California, and author of *Healthy Homestyle Cooking*. "Or fold them into an egg-white omelette," she says.

• Don't add mushrooms in the early stages of preparing a cooked dish, advises Connie Diekman, R.D., a dietitian in St. Louis and a spokesperson for the American Dietetic Association; they can become tough and flavorless. "Add mushrooms toward the end of cooking," she says. "You'll still get the flavor of the raw mushrooms, and they'll be slightly tender."

• Add finely diced mushrooms to tomato sauce, suggests Tribole.

"If you chop them very finely, they actually take on the texture of ground beef," she says.

- For a unique main dish, serve grilled portobello mushrooms, suggests Mona Sutnick, R.D., Ed.D., a dietitian in Philadelphia and a spokesperson for the American Dietetic Association. "Portobellos are a meaty sort of mushroom, and their caps are four to seven inches across," she says. "A restaurant in Philadelphia grills them and serves them with polenta and herbs."

～✻～

NIACIN

The Right Dose Can Make a Difference

Looking for a pill that lowers LDL ("bad") cholesterol, increases HDL ("good") cholesterol, drops triglycerides, and costs less than other cholesterol-lowering drugs? "Niacin does all the right things," says David Capuzzi, M.D., Ph.D., director of the Cardiovascular Disease Prevention Center at Thomas Jefferson University Hospital in Philadelphia.

These "right things," studies show, are niacin's double-digit impact on all of the above, when taken in doses of about 1,000 to 3,000 milligrams daily. That's 50 to 150 times higher than the Daily Value for niacin, a B vitamin that's found in small quantities in food. At those levels, however, niacin is a prescription drug, not a food supplement.

Also known as nicotinic acid or vitamin B_3, niacin has a bad reputation that stems in part from a highly publicized 1994 study. That study concluded that serious liver side effects were common with niacin. However, those researchers used higher-than-recommended doses. More recent research has shown that proper doses lead to infrequent liver complications. Still, if your doctor prescribes niacin, he will monitor your liver enzymes so that the dose can be modified or discontinued at the first sign of any trouble. Other side effects of niacin may include gout and high blood sugar, so it may not be prescribed if you have high uric acid levels (which cause gout) or diabetes.

The other big reason doctors have snubbed niacin is its most common side effect. People who take it often experience flushing, similar to a hot flash. It's like a mild sunburn that usually occurs in the face and sometimes in the chest. This unpleasant effect usually subsides as your body gets used to the drug. Research shows that flushing also can be eliminated 80 percent of the time by taking niacin with meals; avoiding alcohol, spicy foods, and hot liquids; and not skipping doses. It may also help to take an aspirin before taking niacin.

Whether taking niacin in supplement form is right for you depends on your cholesterol profile. Never start taking large doses of niacin on your own. Instead, check with your doctor.

OATS

Brimming Bowls of Goodness

Remember the oat bran craze of the late 1980s? Reacting to several encouraging medical studies—and resulting newspaper headlines—cholesterol-conscious people began eating oat bran by the bowlful. Food manufacturers, reacting to our sudden enthusiasm for all things oat bran, added it to just about everything. (Some bakeries were even selling oat bran doughnuts!)

Then, as suddenly as it began, it seemed, our oat bran mania died, a casualty of more headlines. This time, they reported, a study had concluded that oat bran is no better at lowering blood cholesterol than white bread.

End of story? No. Oats do appear to cause a modest reduction in blood cholesterol, and experts say that oats can be a valuable part of a low-fat diet. But when it comes to lowering blood cholesterol, no one food is a magic bullet. Eating a diet low in fat—especially saturated fat—is still one of the best ways to lower your blood cholesterol, say experts.

Stick with It

Oats contain lots of soluble fiber, the kind proven to reduce "bad" LDL cholesterol. "When you cook oats, they're sticky," says Kay Stanfill, R.D., adjunct assistant professor in the Department of Nutritional Sciences at the University of Oklahoma Health Sciences Center in Oklahoma City. "That sticky, gelatinous matter is soluble fiber."

Barley, beans and many fruits and vegetables also contain soluble fiber. But there is something unique about oats' cholesterol-busting ability, says James W. Anderson, M.D., professor of medicine and clinical nutrition at the University of Kentucky College of Medicine in Lexington and author of *Dr. Anderson's High-Fiber Fitness Plan.* "While oat bran and beans have roughly equivalent overall cholesterol-lowering effects, oat bran preserves HDL cholesterol (the 'good' kind) a little better," he says.

The Proof Is in the Porridge

Researchers have conducted a number of studies on the association between consuming oat bran and lower blood cholesterol levels. Investigators at Northwestern University Medical School in Chicago divided 80 men and women with high cholesterol into two groups. The first group ate two servings (about two ounces per serving) of instant oats a day. The second group stuck to their normal eating habits. After eight weeks, the oat group's total cholesterol had declined by about 15 milligrams/deciliter.

At the University of Kentucky College of Medicine, 20 men with high cholesterol consumed diets supplemented with either oat bran or wheat bran, both of which were added to cereal and muffins. After three weeks, the total cholesterol of the men eating oat bran had fallen 12.8 percent, and their LDL cholesterol had declined 12.1 percent. The men who consumed wheat bran saw no such declines in cholesterol.

In an attempt to summarize the existing research on oat bran and cholesterol, researchers from all over the world, including the United States, pooled data from ten studies and 1,300 people. The researchers found that people who ate three grams a day of the soluble fiber found in oat bran (equal to about 1⅓ bowls of oat bran cereal) saw their blood cholesterol fall an average of nearly six milligrams/deciliter in three months or less. What's more, those who began with the highest cholesterol readings (230 milligrams/deciliter or more) experienced the greatest decreases in blood cholesterol—an average decline of 16 milligrams/deciliter.

Five Ways to Feel Your Oats

Want to add oat bran to your diet? These tips can help.

• Choose a whole oat product, advises Stanfill. "Look for the words 'rolled oats,' 'steel-cut oats,' 'Irish oats' or 'oat bran,'" she says. Instant oatmeal probably isn't a whole oat product, she adds.

• Top a bowl of oat bran or oatmeal with a low-fat, low-cholesterol topping such as fat-free milk, fresh fruit or even a dollop or two of fat-free flavored yogurt.

• Try adding a small amount of oat bran to other dishes, suggests Dr. Anderson. "You can mix oat bran or oatmeal into ground-meat dishes, casseroles and pancakes," he says.

• Bake your own oat bran muffins using low-fat ingredients, including fat-free milk, egg substitute and unsaturated oil instead of butter. Try using ¾ cup of oat bran for every ¼ cup of flour in a 12-muffin recipe. For extra-tasty muffins, try adding a small amount of crushed pineapple to the mix, suggests Dr. Anderson.

Be wary of store-bought oat bran muffins. "They can contain a lot of fat," says Robert J. Nicolosi, Ph.D., director of the Cardiovascular Disease Control Center at the University of Lowell in Massachusetts. "The ideal way to get fiber is through grains and cereals."

• Don't expect a bowl of oat bran to compensate for a fat-laden diet. "All of the soluble fiber in the world isn't going to compensate for eating too much saturated fat," notes Linda Van Horn, R.D., Ph.D., associate professor of preventive medicine at Northwestern University Medical School.

~❧~

OLIVE OIL

The Leading Good-for-You Fat

Olive oil: golden essence of the Mediterranean. Nectar of the gods. Cholesterol crusher.

This fragrant oil, touted by the great Greek physician Hippocrates as a natural remedy over 2,000 years ago, is brimming with monounsaturated fat, which tends to cut heart-threatening LDL cholesterol while it preserves—or even raises—heart-saving HDL cholesterol. One study suggests that the monounsaturated fat in olive oil may actually change the chemical composition of HDL cholesterol, making it better at routing LDL. No wonder some heart experts have recommended substituting olive oil for the artery-clogging saturated fat that plagues the typical American diet.

But make no mistake: Drowning your food in olive oil will not protect your heart from the ravages of ribs, french fries and rocky road ice cream, maintain experts. Too much of any fat—even monounsaturated fat—can wreak havoc on your cholesterol level, not to mention your waistline.

The good news is, a little bit of olive oil yields a lot of flavor. What's more, you're likely to find that this golden oil tastes delicious on everything from corn on the cob to crusty peasant bread. Here's how to "Mediterraneanize" your menu and help protect your heart.

The Mediterranean Miracle

Not surprisingly, people in the Mediterranean region, where most olive oil is produced and enthusiastically consumed, have reaped the greatest health benefits from olive oil—a phenomenon first proven by Ancel Keys, Ph.D., professor emeritus of public health in the School of Public Health at the University of Minnesota in Minneapolis. In the Seven Countries Study—a seminal study dating back to the 1950s—Keys discovered that while Italian, Greek and other Mediterranean men consumed almost as much dietary fat as Americans, they consumed most of that fat in the form of olive oil. Keys associated the Mediterraneans' consumption of monounsaturated fat, particularly olive oil, with their lower rates of heart disease.

More recent studies have reached similar conclusions about the cholesterol-busting powers of olive oil. Researchers at the Universidad Autonoma de Madrid in Spain had 21 pre- and postmenopausal women follow a high-fat diet for four months. For the first month of the study, the women ate a diet high in saturated fat (such as butter) and lower in polyunsaturated and monounsaturated fats. For the next six weeks, the women followed an olive oil–rich diet lower in saturated and polyunsaturated fats. And for six weeks after that, the women consumed a diet rich in sunflower oil (a polyunsaturated fat) and lower in monounsaturated and saturated fats.

The women's total and LDL cholesterol fell on both the olive oil and sunflower oil diets. But their HDL cholesterol increased only on the olive oil diet—and fell on the sunflower oil diet.

In another study, researchers at the University of Nijmegen in the Netherlands had 48 healthy people follow a high-fat diet. Then for five weeks, half of these folks followed a low-fat diet (22 percent of calories from fat). The other half consumed a high-fat diet (41 percent of calories from fat), but the fat came mostly from monounsaturates such as olive oil.

After a month, both groups' total cholesterol had fallen. But the HDL cholesterol of the folks on the low-fat diet had declined an average of 7.3 milligrams/deciliter, while HDL had actually increased 1.1 milligrams/deciliter in the people who followed the olive oil program.

An Olive Oil Primer

When it comes to olive oil, a little goes a long way. "Compared with some other oils, olive oil is so flavorful that you can use less of it," says Barbara Levine, R.D., Ph.D., associate clinical professor of nutrition in medicine at Cornell University Medical College in New York City.

Olive oil connoisseurs categorize the flavor of olive oil as mild (with a light or buttery taste), semifruity (a stronger, more olivelike flavor) or fruity (oil with an intense olive flavor). And despite what you may

---

VERSIONS OF VIRGINS

When it comes to olive oil, "refined" isn't a compliment. Confused? Relax: This guide can help you decipher the labels and select the perfect oil.

Extra-virgin olive oil. Produced in limited quantities, extra-virgin oil is the best and most expensive grade of olive oil that money can buy. Most people use extra-virgin oil, which has an intense fruity or peppery flavor, to flavor foods after they've been cooked rather than as a cooking oil.

Virgin olive oil. The flavor of this oil isn't as perfect as that of extra-virgin oil and is slightly more acidic.

Olive oil. Most people use this blend of refined and virgin oils for cooking.

"Light" olive oil. Perfect for baking, this extra-refined oil has little or no olive taste. But don't be fooled: Light olive oil contains the same amount of fat and calories as other oils.

---

have heard, the color of olive oil has nothing to do with its flavor. Like wine, olive oil gets its unique color, flavor and aroma from the olives used and the climate and soil conditions in which they were grown. So you may want to taste-test olive oil to find the variety and brand most pleasing to your palate.

Here's how to get more olive oil into your diet.

• Spread crusty bread with olive oil rather than butter, suggests Dr. Levine. Or rub a toasted slice of bread with a piece of garlic, then drizzle the bread with olive oil.

• Dress salads the Mediterranean way—with a small amount of extra-virgin olive oil and a little bit of vinegar, suggests Gene A. Spiller, D.Sc., Ph.D., director of the Health Research and Studies Center in Los Altos, California, and author of *The Superpyramid Eating Program.*

• Brush corn on the cob with extra-virgin olive oil rather than butter or margarine, suggests Dr. Spiller.

• Add olive oil to sauces, marinades and any other dish in which you want a more robust flavor, says Tammy Baker, R.D., a nutritionist in Cave Creek, Arizona, and a spokesperson for the American Dietetic Association. You might bathe fresh garlic and spinach with a small amount of olive oil spray and sauté in a nonstick skillet, suggests Lynn Fischer, author of *Healthy Indulgences*. Spinach-lovers will enjoy this Sicilian-style dish, says Fischer.

• Bake or sauté fish in olive oil rather than butter, says Dr. Levine. "Olive oil expands in the pan, so you need much less of it," she says.

• Bake with olive oil. Yes, you read right. "People in Italy bake magnificent desserts with olive oil," says Dr. Levine. "You can substitute olive oil for butter, margarine or vegetable shortening in cakes,

Heart-Healthy ♡
Indulgences

EXTRA-VIRGIN OLIVE OIL: WORTH THE EXTRA $$$

Some things in life cost more than others. In the case of extra-virgin olive oil, the added expense is worth it, since studies show that the oil will benefit your health.

Researchers in Spain (where use of olive oil is widespread) asked 24 men to prepare meals with either refined or extra-virgin olive oil. After 3 months, the experts concluded that extra-virgin oil was more effective than regular olive oil at stopping the men's LDL cholesterol from oxidizing. Researchers think that white blood cells pick up only oxidized LDL and deposit it in artery linings; thus, since extra-virgin oil contains high levels of antioxidants, it may help slow plaque formation in the arteries (atherosclerosis).

The good news doesn't stop there. A study in Greece showed that people with the lowest lifetime consumption of extra-virgin olive oil had a $2\frac{1}{2}$ times greater chance of developing rheumatoid arthritis than those with the highest consumption. Rheumatologist Hayes Wilson, M.D., spokesperson for the Arthritis Foundation, says, "If you have rheumatoid arthritis in your family and want to take every possible step to protect yourself, you might try adding olive oil to your diet." And, he adds, since the type of oil consumed in Greece is extra-virgin, that may offer additional protection.

While all four standard grades of olive oil—extra-virgin, virgin, pure and extra-light—are high in heart-healthy monounsaturated fats, extra-virgin is best because it's made from the first pressing of the olives (with acid levels under 1 percent). The other grades, while still good for you, are generally more acidic and processed.

pies and other desserts." She suggests using a light variety, "so you won't taste olive oil in your dessert."

• Don't cook with extra-virgin olive oil, advises Dr. Levine. "Heating this oil will accomplish only what's called perfuming the kitchen," she says. "That is, the olive oil goes into the air rather than into the food. Save extra-virgin oil for salads or for drizzling over pasta."

Before You Get All Oiled Up

Don't forget that olive oil is still 100 percent fat and contains 120 calories per tablespoon. So overusing olive oil may cause you to gain weight—not a heart-smart move, say experts.

"Many people are drowning their foods in olive oil, thinking that they're doing themselves a service," says Karen Miller Kovach, R.D., chief nutritionist at Weight Watchers International in Jericho, New York. But it's better to substitute olive oil for saturated fats such as butter, says Kovach, than to add olive oil to an already high-fat diet.

Dr. Levine agrees. "Don't consume lots of olive oil or any other kind of oil. Anoint your food with a small amount of olive oil, like the Italians do."

See also Mediterranean Diet

ONIONS

The Benefits of a Good Cry

Sure, chopping onions may bring tears to your eyes or start your nose running like a leaky faucet. But those tears and sniffles might be worth it: The same compounds in onions that leave many of us helplessly weepy-eyed may also help wallop elevated blood cholesterol and bust up blood clots that can trigger a heart attack.

There's not yet conclusive proof that onions can help control cholesterol or prevent a heart attack. But investigators continue to be intrigued by the potential health benefits of this odoriferous bulb. In one study, researchers in India had ten men consume $3\frac{1}{2}$ ounces of butter a day, which increased their cholesterol levels. The researchers then added about 2 ounces of juice from raw onions to the men's daily servings of butter. The onion extract prevented the expected rise in cholesterol from the butter. It also increased the men's clot-busting activity almost 16 percent, reducing their risk of heart attacks.

Another Indian study found that cholesterol levels were lowest among people who consumed over 600 grams of onions and 50 grams of garlic a week and highest among people who never touched the stuff.

Researchers in the Netherlands found that antioxidant constituents called flavonoids—found in many fruits and vegetables, including onions, tea and apples—reduced the risk of coronary heart disease and heart attack in elderly men, apparently by blocking the formation of clotting compounds in the blood and by interfering with the oxidation of "bad" LDL cholesterol, which leads to the buildup of plaque in the coronary arteries.

Mild-Mannered Onion Power

Many people love the taste and smell of onions. But if you'd like to tone down their taste—or at least dry up your tears as you slice them—these tips are for you.

• Investigate sweet onions, suggests Connie Diekman, R.D., a dietitian in St. Louis and a spokesperson for the American Dietetic Association. There are several varieties of these mild-tasting onions, such as Vidalia, Walla Walla, Maui and Texas Spring Sweet. "Some people even eat them plain," says Diekman.

• Don't fry onions in oil or butter. Instead, "sauté" them in the microwave, suggests Barbie Casselman, a nutrition consultant in Toronto. Place a sliced onion in a microwave-safe bowl, along with a tablespoon or two of water. Cover the bowl with a plate. Then nuke the covered bowl for three to four minutes. "The onions will be as soft as if they had been sautéed in butter," says Casselman.

• To avoid shedding tears as you slice an onion, "hold it under cold water as you cut," suggests Diekman. Or refrigerate the bulb before you slice it, suggests Mona Sutnick, R.D., Ed.D., a dietitian in Philadelphia and a spokesperson for the American Dietetic Association. They're less pungent when they're chilled first, she says.

~✿~

ORANGE JUICE

A Glass or Two Is Good for Your Heart

One of the easiest things you can to do lower your cholesterol is to drink some OJ every day, according to a study by researchers at the University of Western Ontario in London, Canada.

After sipping first one, then two, then three glasses of orange juice a day for four weeks, 25 men and women with relatively high cholesterol levels benefited in two ways: Their HDL cholesterol (the kind that sweeps away artery-clogging fat) levels shot up 21 percent, and their LDL cholesterol levels (the kind that clogs arteries) dropped 16 percent. These preliminary results are remarkable for another reason, since it is normally difficult to change HDL levels through diet, says Elzbieta Kurowska, Ph.D., the study's lead author and research associate at the University of Western Ontario.

"We're not completely sure why orange juice raised HDL," she says, "but we know that it contains hesperidin, a flavonoid less common in other citrus fruits," Flavonoids are the naturally occurring compounds found in many fruits and vegetables, including citrus juices.

The study was small, and there's a possible delay in the effect of the juice, so it's hard to say how many glasses to drink each day. "People with high total cholesterol and low HDL cholesterol could try more orange juice in their diet to see whether it improves their cholesterol profile," Dr. Kurowska advises. (While eating whole oranges has other benefits, it's not a practical way to try to lower your cholesterol, since it takes about four medium oranges to make one glass of juice.)

Since orange juice is high in calories (110 calories per eight ounces), study participants were advised to eat less of other foods to allow for the juice's calories. To reap the potential benefits without adding excess calories, split your daily ration of OJ by mixing four ounces with seltzer for midmorning and midafternoon pick-me-ups.

PECTIN

The Fiber King

You may know it as the stuff that puts the jell in jelly. But pectin—a gummy substance found in most fruits and many vegetables—can help wallop elevated cholesterol as well, say experts.

There are two kinds of fiber: soluble and insoluble. Soluble fiber has been proven to help trounce blood cholesterol.

"Like other types of soluble fiber, pectin has the capacity to reduce blood cholesterol levels," says Thomas Bersot, M.D., associate professor of medicine at the University of California, San Francisco. "Pectin may interfere with the body's absorption of cholesterol, which helps lower blood cholesterol levels."

Pectin may also affect certain enzymes in the liver that produce cholesterol, says James J. Cerda, M.D., professor of medicine at the University of Florida College of Medicine in Gainesville.

"The more pectin you eat, the less cholesterol is produced by the liver," says Dr. Cerda.

Staging a Plaque Attack

In one study, Dr. Cerda and his colleagues had 27 people considered to be at moderate to high risk for coronary heart disease consume either 15 grams of pectin each day (in capsule form) or a placebo each day for a month. Then for another four weeks, the people consuming the pectin took the placebos, and vice versa.

Researchers found that when these folks consumed the pectin supplements as opposed to the placebos, their total cholesterol dropped an average of 7.6 percent, and their "bad" LDL cholesterol plummeted about 10.8 percent.

In another study led by Dr. Cerda, 14 miniature pigs were fed a high-fat diet for more than a year—long enough for the pigs to develop plaque-clogged coronary arteries. Then for another nine months, half of the pigs continued on this same fatty diet plus 3 percent grapefruit pectin. The remaining seven pigs were fed the same diet but with no added pectin.

After nine months, the pectin had not significantly lowered the pigs' cholesterol levels. But the pectin had stopped the progression of, or reduced the extent of, the plaque buildup in the animals' coronary arteries and aortas. In fact, the coronary arteries of the swine who hadn't consumed pectin had narrowed an average of 45 percent, while the arteries of the pectin-fed pigs had narrowed only 24 percent.

Getting Your Peck of Pectin

How much pectin might you have to eat to help send your cholesterol level south? A lot. "The therapeutic dose for water-soluble fibers such as pectin is 15 grams a day," says Dr. Cerda.

Here's how to get more pectin into your diet.

• Load up on fruits and veggies. Pectin-rich vegetables include carrots, lettuce, spinach, beets, brussels sprouts, cabbage, potatoes, onions and peas. Pectin-rich fruits include grapefruit, oranges, bananas, strawberries, peaches, apples, grapes and plums.

• Eat more grapefruit. Whether red, white or pink, grapefruit is one of the best sources of pectin around, suggests Dr. Cerda. "It's also high in vitamin C," he says.

• Eat the whole fruit or vegetable rather than drink its juice, suggests Martin Yadrick, R.D., a dietitian in Manhattan Beach, California, and spokesperson for the American Dietetic Association.

"Juice doesn't contain as much fiber as the fruit itself," says Yadrick. Bonus: You'll most likely feel more satisfied after eating a grapefruit or an apple than after downing a glass of juice.

See also Apples, Carrots

~❧~

POLYUNSATURATED FAT
Moderation (As Usual) Is the Key

If you're trying to lower your cholesterol, your doctor has probably already advised you to replace artery-clogging saturated fat, found primarily in animal products such as red meat and dairy foods, with unsaturated fat, found mostly in plant foods. There are two types of unsaturated fat: monounsaturated, which is abundant in olive oil, canola oil, nuts and avocados, and polyunsaturated, which is found in corn oil, sunflower oil and safflower oil. The American Heart Association recommends that Americans consume no more than 10 percent of their calories from polyunsaturated fat.

Both monounsaturates and polyunsaturates lower "bad" LDL cholesterol. But polyunsaturates tend to lower "good" HDL cholesterol, too. So you may wonder: If polyunsaturates lower the good along with the bad, is it better to opt for monos over polys?

Most doctors endorse unsaturated fat over saturated fat, period. "In general, highly polyunsaturated oils lower LDL cholesterol slightly better than monounsaturated oils," says Robert J. Nicolosi, Ph.D., director of the Cardiovascular Disease Control Center at the University of Lowell in Massachusetts. "But monounsaturated fat is a bit better at preventing reductions in HDL cholesterol. So it's somewhat of a wash. But it's fair to say that you should replace saturated fat with either monounsaturated fat or polyunsaturated fat."

Other doctors echo Dr. Nicolosi's assertion. "One reason that total and LDL cholesterol levels have declined in the United States in the past 30 years is that we're eating less saturated fat and more polyunsaturated fat," says Robert Rosenson, M.D., director of the Preventive Cardiology Center at Rush–Presbyterian–St. Luke's Medical Center in Chicago. What's more, says Dr. Rosenson, declines in HDL cholesterol that are associated with polyunsaturated fat may be more significant in people with low HDL cholesterol than in those with normal or high HDL cholesterol.

Studies comparing the effects of monounsaturates and polyunsaturates are continuing. In the meantime, follow the Golden Rule of cholesterol reduction: Consume all fats in moderation.

"If you replace the saturated fat you get from animal products—such as meat and dairy foods—with unsaturated fat from plants and

ALL POLYS ARE NOT CREATED EQUAL

Some oils with polyunsaturated fats, such as soybean, safflower, grapeseed and corn oils, contain omega-6 fatty acids, which hinder the benefits of omega-3's when consumed in excess. Your best bet is to use them sparingly and focus on oils high in monounsaturated fats and omega-3's, along with varying amounts of vitamin E (an antioxidant that is also considered beneficial to heart health).

OILS	MONO- UNSATURATES (%)	POLY- UNSATURATES (%)	SATURATES (%)	OMEGA-3 FATTY ACIDS (%)
TOP CHOICES				
Hazelnut	82	10.0	8.0	0
Olive	77	9.0	14	0.63
Canola	62	31	7.0	9.73
Peanut	48	34	18.0	0
Sesame	42.0	43.0	15.0	0.3
Walnut	24.0	66.0	10.0	10.92
Flaxseed	21.0	68.0	11.0	55.8
USE OCCASIONALLY*				
Corn	25.0	62.0	13.0	0.73
Soybean	24.0	61.0	15.0	7.1
Grapeseed	17.0	73.0	10.0	0.1
AVOID				
Coconut	6.0	2.0	92.0	0

SOURCE: USDA NUTRIENT DATABASE

*Safflower and sunflower oils should also be used only occasionally, but actual values vary from manufacturer to manufacturer. Check labels for nutrition information.

vegetables, you'll be in good shape," says Christopher Gardner, Ph.D., of the Stanford Center for Research in Disease Prevention at Stanford University Medical Center, who did a comprehensive review of research comparing monounsaturated and polyunsaturated fat and their relative effects on cholesterol levels. "When it comes to HDL and LDL cholesterol levels, it doesn't matter whether the fats are monounsaturated or polyunsaturated, as long as they're not saturated."

See also Canola Oil, Monounsaturated Fat, Olive Oil

POPCORN

The Four-Star Snack

Ever wonder what makes popcorn pop?

The secret lies inside the popcorn kernel itself. When the kernel is exposed to heat, the moisture inside it begins to soften the starch within. As the internal temperature of each kernel rises, this moisture turns to steam and causes the kernel to explode, forcing the starch to expand. Voilà—the kernel bursts into a fluffy piece of popped corn.

That ping-ping-ping of kernels against saucepan lid, air popper or microwaveable bag will be heard billions of times in the United States this year. In an average year, we eat 18 billion quarts of popcorn!

Prepared in a heart-healthy manner, popcorn is a perfect antidote to a snack attack. "It's a high-carbohydrate, low-calorie and filling snack," says Karen Vartan, R.D., a dietitian in Chicago. What's more, half of the fiber in popcorn is soluble, the kind that can help knock points off your blood cholesterol level.

But popcorn is only as healthful as the way it's prepared. "Air-popped popcorn is the way to go," advises Lisa Lauri, R.D., nutrition consultant at North Shore University Hospital in Manhasset, New York.

A typical serving (three cups) of air-popped popcorn contains 81 calories and just a trace of fat. Popcorn popped in oil and drenched in butter or margarine and salt, on the other hand, contains large amounts of total and saturated fat and sodium. So do many varieties of microwaveable and prepopped, ready-to-eat popcorn.

But more than a few of us believe that unless popcorn is bathed in butter and soaked with salt . . . well, it's just not popcorn. "There are two kinds of popcorn-eaters," says Vartan. "The first kind thinks that air-popped popcorn with nothing on it tastes perfectly acceptable. The second kind eats popcorn as a pleasure food, complete with butter or even chocolate. This kind of popcorn is as much a treat as premium ice cream." While there's nothing wrong with treating yourself to gourmet popcorn occasionally, says Vartan, indulging too often can help launch your intake of artery-clogging fat into orbit.

Flavor without Fat

Here's how to make home-popped popcorn extra delicious and how to select heart-smart microwaveable or ready-to-eat popcorn.

• To add pizzazz to air-popped corn, lightly spray it with a vegetable oil cooking spray, such as Pam, and get creative with the seasonings. "Sprinkle the popcorn with some low-fat cheese—perhaps low-fat Cheddar, Monterey Jack or Swiss—along with some caraway or mustard seeds," suggests Vartan.

Other options? "Try sprinkling popcorn with Butter Buds, oregano, basil or sage," suggests Janet Lepke, R.D., a dietitian in Santa Monica, California, and a spokesperson for the American Dietetic Association.

• It's probably not the first popcorn topping that comes to mind, but Vartan suggests coating air-popped corn with dry sugar-free gelatin. "Spray the popcorn lightly with Pam, sprinkle on the gelatin and bake for five minutes at 350°," she says.

• If you buy microwaveable or ready-to-eat popcorn, opt for "light" varieties; they contain less fat and sodium. Many brands, including Orville Redenbacher's, Jolly Time and Pop-Secret, offer lower-fat products as well as their regular lines. Light popcorn isn't necessarily low-fat, however, so check the label for grams of fat and the percentage of calories from fat.

Take note of the serving size, too. "Many people think that a bag is one serving, but each serving might actually be three cups," says Lauri. "There could be nine cups in a bag." So if you munch beyond the first three cups, you may be consuming more fat than you think.

• If you must pop your popcorn in oil, opt for canola oil. But make no mistake: Even popcorn popped in canola oil contains fat, notes Martin Yadrick, R.D., a dietitian in Manhattan Beach, California, and a spokesperson for the American Dietetic Association. "You'll consume less saturated fat if you use canola oil, but you'll still consume fat," says Yadrick. "So the trick is to use less oil when you make popcorn—or, even better, to air-pop."

Pass on Movie Popcorn

If you're like a lot of people, watching the latest blockbuster without a big tub of buttered popcorn is just about unthinkable. But a few years ago, a study conducted by the Center for Science in the Public Interest (CSPI) painted a picture of movie popcorn more frightening than the latest version of *Jurassic Park*.

The CSPI study found that a large tub of butter-flavored popcorn popped in coconut oil, which is 86 percent saturated fat, contains over 1,600 calories and nearly 130 grams of fat. That's as much fat as in eight Big Macs! Even a small tub (about five cups) of butter-flavored popcorn popped in coconut oil packs about 20 grams of fat total, 14 of them saturated.

Most likely, the "butter" is partially hydrogenated soybean oil, which is full of saturated fat and trans fat, an unsaturated fat that raises cholesterol. The good news is, more and more movie chains are offering air-popped corn or are popping popcorn in canola oil. This unsaturated fat is easier on your coronary arteries than the more commonly used coconut oil, a highly saturated fat.

Why do most theaters use coconut oil? People seem to prefer it, says Yadrick. Also, coconut oil has a longer shelf life than unsaturated fats such as canola and corn oils, which may make coconut oil a more attractive choice to theater owners.

To avoid movie popcorn's sat-fat attack, consider taking your own air-popped corn to the theater. You might also suggest that the theater offer air-popped corn as well as the oil-popped kind. You never know.

~❧~

PSYLLIUM

This Natural Laxative Has Other Powers

If you're like most people, you've taken a laxative now and then to get things moving again. But did you know that an ingredient in some laxatives can help lower blood cholesterol?

It's true: Several studies have shown that psyllium, an ingredient in some bulk-forming laxatives, can reduce moderately elevated blood cholesterol. That's because psyllium, derived from the seed husks of a plant with origins in India, is rich in soluble fiber, a gummy substance found in certain fruits and vegetables that has been shown to deflate cholesterol.

"Psyllium is a very good source of soluble fiber," says James W. Anderson, M.D., professor of medicine and clinical nutrition at the University of Kentucky College of Medicine in Lexington and author of *Dr. Anderson's High-Fiber Fitness Plan.* You'll find psyllium in supplement form, such as powders and wafers, as well as in some breakfast cereals.

Taking psyllium supplements to lower cholesterol may not be right for everyone. (More on that in a bit.) But generally speaking, teaming psyllium with a low-fat, low-cholesterol diet can help deflate total and "bad" LDL cholesterol.

Psyllium Solutions

How does psyllium work? Some studies suggest that like other forms of soluble fiber, psyllium prevents the body from reabsorbing a digestive secretion called bile. If the small intestine contains soluble fiber, bile—which contains cholesterol—gets trapped in this gummy stuff and is excreted from the body. Without soluble fiber, the body reabsorbs bile and recycles the cholesterol it contains.

At the University of Kentucky, Dr. Anderson and his colleagues had 44 people following a low-fat, low-cholesterol diet eat either a psyllium-enriched breakfast cereal containing 2.9 grams of psyllium and

3 grams of soluble fiber per serving or a wheat bran cereal containing negligible amounts of soluble fiber. After six weeks, LDL cholesterol dropped nearly 13 percent in the people who ate the psyllium-enriched cereal but only 2.5 percent in the wheat bran group.

Researchers at the University of Cincinnati and Washington University School of Medicine in St. Louis put 118 people with elevated cholesterol (220 milligrams/deciliter or higher) on either a low-fat or a high-fat diet. Some of the participants consumed five grams of psyllium (in sugar-free orange-flavored Metamucil) twice a day, just before breakfast and dinner. The others were given a placebo. After two months on the psyllium, LDL cholesterol fell 7.2 percent in those following the low-fat diet and 6.4 percent in those on the high-fat diet. The LDL cholesterol of the people who took the placebo didn't change.

The Cereal Ingredient That Surprises Some

As mentioned, you can take psyllium as a powder mixed with water or juice, in wafer form or in a psyllium-containing breakfast cereal such as Bran Buds or FiberWise. "Bran Buds are a good choice," says Dr. Anderson. "They contain wheat bran, an insoluble fiber that promotes regularity and health of the colon, as well as soluble fiber, which lowers cholesterol."

If you choose to try a psyllium supplement, follow the recommended dosage on the label, advises Dr. Anderson. Also, for maximum effect, take psyllium with meals. In a study at the University of Toronto, people with mildly high cholesterol who ate Bran Buds for two weeks (1/3 cup at breakfast and 1/3 cup at dinner) saw their cholesterol drop by 8 percent. But people who took psyllium powder, mixed with water, between meals had only a minor drop in cholesterol.

Note: There are some instances in which you should not consume this fiber. Don't use psyllium if you're taking certain prescription drugs. Too much psyllium can slow the absorption of heart medication and blood pressure medication, says Dr. Anderson.

Also, if you've had an allergic reaction to laxatives—or if you have any kind of allergy at all—consult your doctor before taking psyllium. This fiber has caused anaphylaxis (a severe allergic reaction) in some people. Such a reaction is rare, however.

~❦~

RED YEAST RICE EXTRACT

Promising but Problematic

Cultivated on rice, red yeast (*Monascus purpureus*) contains natural substances that are chemically similar to the active ingredients in statin drugs that are widely prescribed for high cholesterol. It appears that these substances, technically known as HMG-CoA reductase inhibitors, stimulate the formation of good (HDL) cholesterol and reduce the production of bad (LDL) cholesterol.

Clinical trials showed that daily consumption of four 600-milligram capsules of a standardized red yeast product called Cholestin produced significant reductions in blood levels of both cholesterol and triglycerides (another blood fat implicated in heart disease).

The first U.S. study of Cholestin involved 83 people with high cholesterol. The 42 who took Cholestin for 12 weeks lowered their total cholesterol by an average of 16 percent. From a total cholesterol level of 250, that's a drop of 40 points.

Cholestin also contains unsaturated fatty acids that appear to lower triglycerides, and at the same time, it appears to increase levels of beneficial HDL cholesterol.

In 1998, the FDA banned over-the-counter sales of Cholestin because it deemed that its active ingredients were too closely related to lovastatin, a prescription drug sold as Mevacor, and therefore infringed on patents for that drug. Pharmanex, the maker of Cholestin, has since been ordered to discontinue sale of the product.

Currently, generic red yeast rice extracts (sometimes called Chinese red yeast) are available. However, these products may be neither safe nor effective. Specific claims for the cholesterol-lowering benefits of generic red yeast rice extract are often based on research on Cholestin, not on the generic supplements.

"A recent analysis found that many of these products, which aren't as well-studied as Cholestin, contain lower levels of the cholesterol-lowering compounds," says Andrew T. Weil, M.D., director of the program in integrative medicine and clinical professor of medicine at the University of Arizona in Tucson and editor of "Dr. Andrew Weil's Self-Healing" newsletter. "Plus, some are contaminated with citrinin, a toxin that causes kidney damage in animals."

Cholestin is less likely to cause liver dysfunction than prescription statin drugs. In the event that it becomes available again, it should be used with caution by anyone with a history of liver disease. For now, generic red yeast extract should also be used cautiously, if at all. It isn't recommended for use by people under 20 or pregnant or nursing women. With so many other safe and effective ways to lower your cholesterol, outlined throughout this book, generic red yeast rice extract may not be worth the risk at this time.

~✤~

SMOKING CESSATION

How to Quit for Good

These days, smoking takes real willpower. If you smoke, chances are you're getting tired of enduring disdainful looks from coworkers who see you standing outdoors on a smoke break. Or you feel frustrated trying to find restaurants that still have smoking sections. But feeling like a social outcast can't begin to match the havoc that smoking can wreak on your cholesterol levels—and the health of your heart. If you need even more reasons to quit, consider these.

• Scientific evidence shows that smoking is a major contributing factor to elevated blood cholesterol and heart disease.
• Smokers tend to have less HDL cholesterol (the "good" kind) and higher total and LDL cholesterol (the "bad" stuff) than nonsmokers.
• Smokers who already have elevated cholesterol are more likely to develop coronary heart disease and suffer heart attacks than nonsmokers are.

Scientists still aren't sure exactly how and why smoking is responsible for elevated cholesterol. To find out, researchers in Turkey studied 58 men (27 who smoked and 31 who did not). They measured the activity of lecithin cholesterol acyltransferase (LCAT), a key factor in shepherding cholesterol to the liver for excretion from the body. The researchers found that smoking affected HDL cholesterol levels in the smokers group and that LCAT activity tended to be lower in smokers than in nonsmokers, suggesting a correlation between smoking and LCAT.

A similar study, conducted by investigators at the University of California, Berkeley, found that the effectiveness of LCAT is "dramatically inhibited" by cigarette smoke. "Cigarette smoke hits human plasma with a double whammy" and reduces both LCAT and HDL, says Mark R. McCall, Ph.D., one of the researchers.

Ground Zero for Your Arteries

Research has shown that smoking damages far more than the lungs; it accelerates hardening of the arteries (arteriosclerosis) and leaves fatty deposits on artery walls (atherosclerosis). Further, cigarette smoke increases the level of carbon monoxide in the blood. This poisonous chemical robs cells of oxygen, injuring the lining of the arteries and allowing fatty material to pass from the bloodstream into the vessel walls.

One study examined the data from 54 earlier studies on the association between smoking and elevated blood cholesterol. This study found that smokers had significantly higher levels of total cholesterol, LDL cholesterol and triglycerides (another blood fat implicated in heart disease), as well as lower levels of HDL cholesterol.

It's Never Too Late to Quit

"If you smoke, quitting is almost certainly the best thing you can do for your cardiovascular system and for your overall health and quality of life," says John W. Zamarra, M.D., founding director of the cardiac rehabilitation program at Placentia-Linda Community Hospital in Brea, California.

There's more good news. Not only is smoking-related damage

reversible, but it *is* possible to quit, no matter how many times you've tried in the past. In fact, one study found that people who can quit for just two weeks are likely to quit for good. More than three million Americans quit smoking every year. So can you—and you'll find lots of help along the way.

Getting Ready to Stop

Quitting smoking isn't easy. But you can make it easier. In one study, researchers from the Arizona Program for Nicotine and Tobacco Research at the University of Arizona in Tucson found that almost two times as many smokers who used buproprion, a prescription antidepressant approved as a smoking cessation aid and sold under the brand name Zyban, were able to abstain from tobacco as those who used either nicotine patches or a placebo (inactive substance). (A nicotine patch delivers enough nicotine through the skin to reduce withdrawal symptoms and help wean you off inhaled smoke that damages your heart and lungs.) The following tips can also help.

• Keep a smoking journal for two weeks before you quit, suggest C. Richard Conti, M.D., and Diana Tonnessen in their book *Beating the Odds against Heart Disease and High Cholesterol.* Jot down the circumstances that most often prompt you to light up: during your coffee break, after dinner, while chatting on the phone, when you're feeling lonely or bored, and so forth.

• After a week, review your journal, pinpointing circumstances that prompt you to smoke. Then list alternatives to smoking during those times. If your journal shows that you tend to smoke after meals, for example, brush your teeth or take a walk instead.

• Decide whether you want to quit smoking all at once—that is, "cold turkey"or taper off. While you may decide to stop smoking gradually, there's evidence that most successful quitters go cold turkey.

• Pick a Quit Day and mark it on your calendar. Make it no later than one week away. Many experts suggest quitting on a weekend, when most people have better control of their time, surroundings and circumstances.

• Get a buddy to help you make it through the quitting process. This person can be a nonsmoker, a former smoker or a smoker who will quit with you. Call your buddy when the going gets rough.

• Tell your family, friends and coworkers about your Quit Day. Let-

PATCHING UP HDL

Sure, quitting smoking can increase "good" HDL cholesterol. But if you're using nicotine transdermal replacement (better known as the nicotine patch) to kick the habit, you may be wondering: Won't using a nicotine patch continue to lower HDL levels? Maybe not, according to one study.

Researchers at the University of Minnesota Medical School in Minneapolis examined the effect of the nicotine patch in people who abstained from smoking. After six weeks, these folks' blood pressure, heart rates and "bad" LDL cholesterol dropped while their HDL cholesterol and triglycerides increased—even while they were using active nicotine patches. But patches aren't magical, experts note. "People who expect nicotine patches to miraculously make them stop smoking will be disappointed," says Gary DeNelsky, Ph.D., director of the smoking cessation program at the Cleveland Clinic Foundation in Ohio. "The patch should be used under a doctor's supervision as part of a comprehensive smoking cessation program."

ting people know about your decision to quit smoking will help hold you to your resolve.

• Call or write your local chapter of the American Heart Association, the American Cancer Society or the American Lung Association and ask for their free brochures and pamphlets on smoking cessation.

• Get some kind of exercise. "Women who work out are conscious of their health and tend not to smoke," says Myra Muramoto, M.D., assistant professor of family and community medicine and medical director of the Arizona Program for Nicotine and Tobacco Research.

A Quit-Day Checklist

Here's what to do when Quit Day dawns.

• Throw away all of your cigarettes and matches. Soak the cigarettes in water so you can't scrounge them out of the trash.
• Hide all the ashtrays. Better yet, get rid of them.
• Lay in a supply of healthy snacks such as celery, carrots, apples, sunflower seeds and air-popped popcorn. They'll keep your mouth and fingers busy without wreaking havoc on your shape.

• Take a long walk or visit a nonsmoking environment such as a library, museum or movie theater.

• Plan to have your teeth cleaned to get rid of tobacco stains. Resolve to keep them that way.

• Avoid stressful situations and smoking environments (bars, for example). Spend as much time as possible in places where smoking isn't permitted.

What about withdrawal symptoms? Well, there's good news and bad news. The bad news first: About 80 percent of smokers experience such symptoms when they quit, from headaches and fatigue to nausea, diarrhea and constipation. Some people also feel anxious, depressed or irritable or have trouble sleeping. The good news: Withdrawal symptoms tend to subside in two to three days, after the nicotine has left your body, and will be gone—or nearly so—within a couple of weeks.

Staying Off 'Em

Most people are capable of quitting smoking. The key is to not start again. Here are three ways to kick the habit for good.

• Be alert for "smoke signals." One study identified the four most likely relapse scenarios: during social drinking, after a meal, while feeling anxious at work and while feeling depressed or anxious when at home alone.

• Learn a relaxation technique, such as deep breathing or progressive relaxation. If smoking helps you relax, "you're likely to feel more stressed when you quit smoking unless you have other ways to manage stress that aren't centered around cigarettes," says Dean Ornish, M.D., president and director of the Preventive Medicine Research Institute in Sausalito, California, and author of *Dr. Dean Ornish's Program for Reversing Heart Disease.*

• On an index card, list two or three of your most important reasons for quitting smoking. Stash the card in your pocket or purse, where you used to keep your cigarettes. Pull it out and go over the list often, particularly when you feel the urge to smoke.

See also Stress Management, Yoga

SOY FOODS

A *"Cult Food" Goes Mainstream*

What a difference a few decades make! Once disdained as bland fare strictly for health nuts, soy milk, soy hot dogs, veggie burgers and other soy products are entering the mainstream. More and more regular folks are quaffing soy beverages, scarfing down soybean-based "meatless" burgers and franks, and discovering how succulent soy foods can be.

And not a moment too soon, it seems. Scientists studying the potential healing properties of soy have discovered a grab bag of health benefits. There's evidence that adding just a small amount of soy to your diet can help fight certain cancers, soothe menopausal symptoms, boost your immune system and, yes, lower blood cholesterol.

In October 1999, the FDA authorized the inclusion on food labels of health claims associated with soy protein and the reduced risk of coronary heart disease. Several studies indicate that a total daily intake of 25 grams of soy protein (the amount in ½ cup of Nutlettes cereal or eight ounces of plain soy milk) as part of a low-fat diet significantly lowers total cholesterol and LDL cholesterol levels. Soybeans are a rich source of isoflavones, a class of phytoestrogens found predominantly in legumes and beans.

People in Asian countries, who tend to consume soy-rich diets, seem to have reaped most of soy's potential health benefits. The Japanese, for example, live longer than any other nationality in the world. What's more, Japanese men have the lowest rate of death from heart disease in the world, and Japanese women have the second lowest. The average Japanese person eats 50 to 80 grams (about two to three ounces) of soy food a day; the typical American eats 5 grams a day.

In one study, Japanese researchers examined the relationship between intake of flavonols, flavones and isoflavones (found in soy) and its effect on blood chemistry. The study participants were 115 women ages 29 to 78. The women's major source of flavonoids was onions, and they got isoflavones from tofu. Their total intake of isoflavones was more than that of other dietary antioxidants, such as flavonoids, carotenoids and vitamin E.

The result: Their total cholesterol and LDL cholesterol levels dropped. The researchers think that since flavonoid and isoflavone intake is significant in Japan that Japanese women's high consumption of those compounds may explain why they have a low incidence of coronary heart disease compared with women in other countries.

You Don't Have to Eat Tofu (Unless You Want To)

Tofu is perhaps the most well known soy food. Like pasta, this soft, mild-tasting substance takes on the flavor of whatever it's cooked with, so it tastes equally good in the spiciest chili and the creamiest cheesecake—and in virtually any other dish.

But if tofu isn't to your liking, you can still enjoy your soy. Today, most supermarkets carry a wide variety of soy beverages, canned or frozen soybeans, soy nuts and commercially prepared soy-based products, from cheese and yogurt to meat analogs (meat substitutes made from soy protein).

Keep in mind, though, that wolfing down tofu or soy-based breakfast "sausage" on top of a burgers-and-fries diet isn't likely to reduce your cholesterol. It works only as part of a low-fat, low-cholesterol diet. And according to experts, replacing a portion of the meat and dairy foods in your diet with their tasty soy impersonators can be a heart-smart move.

The Joy of Soy

Why does soy send cholesterol south? Experts aren't sure. One likely reason is that soy foods, while moderately high in fat, are still lower in fat—particularly artery-choking saturated fat—than meat and dairy products. So replacing animal protein with protein from soy products would theoretically lower blood cholesterol. "Soybeans also are fairly high in fiber," says Kristi A. Steinmetz, Ph.D., consulting nutritional epidemiologist in the Division of Epidemiology at the University of Minnesota in Minneapolis. "This could explain the lowering effect on blood cholesterol."

There are other theories, too. Some investigators speculate that a

HOW TO SPEAK SOY

Don't know tofu from tempeh? Relax—this primer can help introduce you to the joy of soy.

Isolated soy protein. A powdered form of soy protein found in powdered weight-loss drinks and other products.

Meat analogs. These soy-based "meats" include cold cuts, bacon, sausage, franks and burgers.

Soy flour. Made by flaking and grinding roasted soybeans. You can replace up to 20 percent of regular flour with soy flour. Also, use defatted soy flour; the regular variety is very high in fat.

Soy milk. A creamy, milk-like drink made from ground soaked soybeans and water. You can drink soy milk straight, pour it over cereal or substitute it for whole or skim milk in other dishes.

Tempeh. Cakes of cooked, fermented soybeans, laced with a mold that gives tempeh its distinctive flavor. Tempeh is usually grilled, roasted, steamed or added to soups.

Texturized soy protein. Made from soy flour, TSP is a meat substitute that is used to replace part or all of the meat in chili or hamburgers. You buy TSP in dry form and add water before use.

Tofu. A creamy white, soft cake made from curded soy milk. Tofu can be sliced, diced or mashed and used in soups, stir-fries, casseroles and sandwiches.

certain substance in soy, genistein, may help keep fatty plaques from clogging the arteries. Like isoflavones, genistein is a phytoestrogen, a type of plant substance that some researchers believe may help prevent certain types of cancer.

Other research suggests that soy may help the liver excrete cholesterol-rich bile acids, which aid in digestion. When the liver replaces these acids, it draws from the cholesterol circulating in the blood. Presto—your blood cholesterol sinks.

"More than 40 studies have shown that soy protein lowers blood cholesterol," says Herbert Pierson, Ph.D., vice-president of Preventive Nutrition Consultants in Woodinville, Wisconsin, and former project director of the Cancer Preventive Designer Food Project at the National Cancer Institute in Rockville, Maryland.

A team of researchers led by James W. Anderson, M.D., professor of medicine and clinical nutrition at the University of Kentucky College

---

A BEGINNER'S GUIDE TO TOFU

Want to give tofu a try? Follow these tips.

• Select low-fat or fat-free tofu. Regular versions can get anywhere from 30 to over 50 percent of their calories from fat.
• Select tofu curded with calcium sulfate. This variety contains 860 milligrams of calcium, compared with 258 milligrams of calcium in tofu curded with nigari (magnesium chloride).
• Buy tofu in sealed packages. Tofu that sits in water and is exposed to the open air has been found to contain high levels of bacteria.

---

of Medicine in Lexington and author of *Dr. Anderson's High-Fiber Fitness Plan*, analyzed 29 separate studies involving a total of 743 people that examined how soy protein affects blood cholesterol. Most of these studies were conducted with isolated soy protein (ISP) or texturized soy protein (TSP). ISP is a powdered form of soy protein and is often used in powdered weight-loss drinks and other products. TSP is a meat substitute made from soy flour and is often found in hot dogs, hamburgers and sausages. You can also buy TSP in dry form.

The investigators found that consuming 47 grams of soy protein per day instead of animal protein lowered total cholesterol by 9.3 percent, "bad" LDL cholesterol by 12.9 percent and triglycerides (another blood fat implicated in heart disease) by 10.5 percent.

Investigators at the University of Illinois at Urbana-Champaign had 25 men with high cholesterol follow a low-fat, low-cholesterol diet. The men were also assigned to one of four groups. For four consecutive four-week periods, the men substituted muffins made with 50 grams of soy protein for half of their normal protein intake. The soy protein came from either soy flour, ISP and soy fiber or ISP alone. (During part of the study, they ate muffins not containing soy.)

The results? The ISP-only muffins lowered the men's total cholesterol by 12 percent and their LDL cholesterol by 11.5 percent. Since every 1 percent drop in total cholesterol results in a 2 percent reduction in the risk of coronary heart disease, these men lowered their risk by 24 percent. Some of the same investigators replicated these results in a later study, showing that even 25 grams of soy protein reduced total cholesterol in 21 men with high cholesterol.

You'll Never Miss the Meat

Look for soy-based products, from tofu (often found in the produce section) to commercially prepared "meat products" such as vegetable burgers in your local supermarket. You'll probably find ISP, TSP and tempeh in health food stores. The following tips can help you enjoy your soy.

• Mix mashed tofu with diced vegetables, herbs and spices and use it as a vegetable dip or sandwich filling.
• Add cubed tofu to stir-fried vegetables.
• Crumble tofu into spaghetti sauce or chili.
• Pour soy milk over cereal or substitute it for whole milk in soups, cakes, puddings and other dishes that call for milk.
• Combine chilled vanilla soy milk and chilled coffee in a frosted mug for a refreshing "iced soy cappuccino."
• Grill sliced tempeh, then top it with regular burger fixings, suggests registered pharmacist Earl Mindell, Ph.D., professor of nutrition at Pacific Western University in Los Angeles and author of *Earl Mindell's Soy Miracle.*
• Add ISP to baked goods.

ᴥᴥᴥ

STRESS MANAGEMENT

The No-Sweat Cure

The hassles and headaches of everyday life eventually catch up with all of us. But stress can give you more than a yen to escape to an as yet undiscovered South Seas island. There's some evidence that chronic stress can elevate cholesterol and set the stage for coronary heart disease.

Fortunately, you can learn to reduce the stress in your life using a variety of simple techniques. What's more, learning to feel challenged by stress rather than overwhelmed by it can further reduce the effect of stress on your health, say experts. In other words, while you can't always control the sources of your stress, you can change the way you react to them.

Not every heart expert believes that stress causes elevated cholesterol. Stress does have an effect on cholesterol levels, although "it's not nearly as important a factor as diet," says Dean Ornish, M.D., president and director of the Preventive Medicine Research Institute in Sausalito, California, and author of *Dr. Dean Ornish's Program for Reversing Heart Disease*. Nevertheless, if you're following a low-fat, low-cholesterol diet and making other lifestyle changes that lower your risk of heart disease, why not give your response to stress a makeover, too? So unclench your jaw, count to ten and explore how keeping your cool might help keep the lid on cholesterol.

The Stone Age Response

Ironically, the same physiological reaction to stress that helped our caveman ancestors outrun predators may play some role in modern man's (and woman's) proclivity for developing coronary heart disease. This reaction, called the fight-or-flight response, is your inborn red-alert system that readies your body to repel a threat—real or imagined.

During the fight-or-flight response, your body releases stress hormones such as cortisol and adrenaline into your bloodstream. These hormones speed up your breathing, increase your heart rate and accelerate the flow of blood to your arms and legs (the better to help you flee). But if your body triggers this inner alarm dozens of times a day, it can lay the foundation for heart disease.

"Stress seems to accelerate the depositing of plaque into the arteries independent of its effect on blood cholesterol," says Dr. Ornish. In other words, he says, the harmful part of stress has less to do with its effect on cholesterol than its effect on the arteries themselves.

"Stress can make your arteries constrict, which can reduce blood

---

AHHHH . . . TRY THIS RELAXING ROUTINE

Stress reduction techniques such as yoga and meditation have been shown to elicit the relaxation response. This physiological state lowers heart and breathing rates, slows brain waves and even lowers blood pressure in some people, according to Herbert Benson, M.D., chief of the Division of Behavioral Medicine at Beth Israel Deaconess Medical Center in Boston, associate professor of medicine at Harvard Medical School and author of *The Relaxation Response*. Here's how to perform a stress reduction technique called progressive relaxation.

1. Get comfortable. You can sit up or lie down, whichever you prefer.
2. Close your eyes.
3. Inhale gently and make a fist with your right hand. Hold the fist for 5 to 7 seconds, exhale and relax. Feel the tension drain from your hand and forearm, comparing the sensations of how your arm feels relaxed and how it feels tense. Rest for about 45 seconds, then repeat a second time.
4. Tense and relax your left hand as you did with your right.
5. Repeat this exercise from your head to your toes, tensing and relaxing each muscle group in the following order: After your hands, tense and relax your biceps, facial muscles (frown, then relax), neck, upper back (pull your shoulders back as though trying to touch them together behind you), chest (try to pull your shoulders in front of you), stomach, thighs and calves.

---

flow to the heart," says Dr. Ornish. "It can cause something called plaque hemorrhage, which is a rupture of the lining of the arteries that can lead to the arteries becoming obstructed. And stress can cause blood to clot faster, which can lead to a heart attack."

Arterial Terrorists: Beef, Butter and . . . Burnout?

Think burgers and butter are your arteries' only enemies? Think again. Years ago, a well-known study demonstrated that accountants' blood cholesterol skyrocketed by as many as 100 points above their usual levels during tax season. Another study showed that students' blood cholesterol spiked during exams. Here are a few other studies linking stress with stratospheric cholesterol counts.

Researchers at the University of Pittsburgh had 44 healthy men and women either take a complicated computerized test to raise their stress levels or rest quietly for 20 minutes. Blood samples were taken before and after the test and the rest period. Those who took the test showed significant increases in total and "bad" LDL cholesterol.

Researchers in Israel studied 104 men between the ages of 24 and 68. These men didn't have cardiovascular disease, but they did have highly stressful jobs and were defined by the researchers as "burned out." (The study defined burnout as a mix of physical fatigue, mental exhaustion and other factors.) After controlling for age, weight and other factors, the researchers discovered that the total cholesterol of the most burned-out men was 14 percent higher than that of the most relaxed men. What's more, the most stressed-out men had significantly higher LDL cholesterol, the kind that wreaks the most cardiovascular damage.

Researchers at the Brown University Program in Medicine in Providence, Rhode Island, drew blood from 114 men and women, then administered two psychological tests used to measure anxiety and responses to it. After factoring in age, weight and smoking habits, the researchers found that men who repressed their feelings tended to have higher cholesterol than men who didn't. Interestingly, women who repressed negative emotions had lower total and LDL cholesterol than women who didn't. One researcher has suggested that emotional stress may exert a lower physiological toll on women than on men.

Learning to Let Go

The bad news: There's no way to avoid stress. The good news: You can cope with stress in a more heart-healthy manner, say experts. "The impact of emotional stress has little to do with what's actually causing the stress and everything to do with how well you tolerate it," says David Bresler, Ph.D., a stress and imagery specialist at the Los Angeles Healing Arts Center. "Some people experience minimal stress and fall apart, while others face serious stress and don't have a problem with it."

So before you come apart at the seams, consider your cholesterol level and try these stress-busting tips.

• Breathe deeply. "Your breathing is a reflection of your mental state. It's a bridge between your mind and your body, and it can be used to change your frame of mind," says Dr. Ornish. "If you're feeling anxious, your breathing becomes more rapid and shallow. But consciously making yourself breathe more slowly and deeply can help calm you."

• Get some real exercise. According to experts, aerobic exercise, such as a brisk stroll, can help reduce the amount of stress-producing hormones barreling through your bloodstream. "Exercise is a great stress-reducing tool," says Peter O. Kwiterovich, Jr., M.D., professor of medicine and director of the Lipid Research and Atherosclerosis Unit at Johns Hopkins University School of Medicine in Baltimore and author of *The Johns Hopkins Complete Guide for Preventing and Reversing Heart Disease.* "I recommend regular aerobic exercise. Try to exercise a half-hour a day, three or four times a week."

• Don't spread yourself too thin—it's a major cause of stress, says James W. Anderson, M.D., professor of medicine and clinical nutrition at the University of Kentucky College of Medicine in Lexington and author of *Dr. Anderson's High-Fiber Fitness Plan.* "Schedule your time carefully and learn to say no when you need to," advises Dr. Anderson.

• Try turning a stressful situation into a challenge, suggests Dr. Bresler. "If your boss demands a report in two hours, for example, you can think 'This isn't fair' or 'I might get fired if I don't do a good job,'" he says. Thinking this way "can trigger fear and anger as well as the physiological responses associated with those emotions," says Dr. Bresler.

But if you choose to think "This is a real challenge! Let's see what I can accomplish in two hours," you can transform negative stress into the positive kind, says Dr. Bresler: "You can wrap the identical situation in a completely different package, which will influence how your body responds." As the saying goes, "Perception is reality."

See also Exercise, Yoga

꧁꧂

TEA

Get It While It's Green

If your day isn't complete without a cup (or two) of tea, you could be doing your heart a favor. Research indicates that tea, especially the variety known as green tea, may help ward off heart disease and reduce blood cholesterol levels.

Tea is the most widely consumed beverage in the world, second only to water. The United States ranks seventh in tea consumption, behind countries such as India and Russia.

Tea leaves are processed in a variety of ways to make three basic types of tea: black, green and oolong. Black tea, the kind that most Americans drink, is fermented—that is, the leaves are partially dried, crushed, allowed to sit for a few hours and then completely dried. Green tea, the variety most often consumed in Japan, Korea and China, is simply steamed, rolled and crushed. Oolong tea, which is partially fermented, is a cross between black and green tea. One cup of tea contains about 27 milligrams of caffeine, about one-third of the amount found in a cup of ground or roasted coffee.

It's green tea that has garnered the most scientific scrutiny—and according to some experts, it may have the most health benefits.

The Muscle behind Tea

Many researchers credit compounds called polyphenols for tea's cardiovascular protection. Polyphenols act as antioxidants, chemicals that help gobble up free radicals—the cell-damaging compounds thought to accelerate aging and play a role in degenerative conditions such as heart disease and cancer. Green tea is bursting with polyphenols. The fermentation process tends to alter or destroy the polyphenols in black and oolong teas, however.

Polyphenols may help hinder the oxidation of "bad" LDL cholesterol, says Robert J. Nicolosi, Ph.D., director of the Cardiovascular Research Center at the University of Lowell in Massachusetts. Oxidation is the chemical process that rusts metal and turns bananas brown and spotty, and it also makes LDL particles more likely to cling to artery walls. Polyphenols may play a role in keeping LDL from accumulating in the coronary arteries, says Dr. Nicolosi. "Polyphenols are reported to be much more active as antioxidants than vitamin E, for example," he says. And one study suggests that the antioxidant properties in tea might also help prevent blood from clotting, which can lead to heart attacks, says Dr. Nicolosi.

Tea also contains flavonoids, antioxidant compounds that seem to short-circuit the process that leads LDL cholesterol to accumulate in the bloodstream. Dutch researchers who conducted a five-year study of 805 men ages 65 to 84 found that the men who ate the most flavonoids (also found in onions, apples and wine) were 50 percent less likely to have a first heart attack and die of heart disease than those who consumed the least.

The Green Scene

Two other studies have found an association between green tea consumption and cholesterol reduction.

Japanese researchers investigated the link between green tea intake and cardiovascular and liver diseases in 1,371 men over age 40. The researchers found that as tea consumption rose, "good" HDL cholesterol increased, while levels of triglycerides (another blood fat implicated in heart disease), total cholesterol and LDL cholesterol fell. In fact, total cholesterol in the men who drank ten or more cups of tea a day was about 6 percent less than in the men who drank three or fewer cups a day.

In another Japanese study of 1,300 men, researchers found that the greater the consumption of green tea, the lower the men's cholesterol. Men who drank two or fewer cups of tea a day had total cholesterol levels averaging 193 milligrams/deciliter. Those who drank between six and eight cups a day had an average cholesterol reading of 188 milligrams/deciliter. And the average cholesterol of men who drank nine or more cups a day was even lower—185 milligrams/deciliter.

Teatime Tips

You want to wallop your blood cholesterol. Should you trade in your coffee mug for a teacup? And how much tea do you need to drink?

Since there is not yet conclusive proof that tea can lower cholesterol, there's no way to know how much tea might do the trick. There's some evidence that drinking a few cups of tea a day may give you a slight edge, however. If you enjoy black tea, avoid adding cream, half-and-half or whole milk, as all are high in fat. Use fat-free or low-fat milk instead. Most people drink green tea without cream or sugar. You can find green tea in some large supermarkets and most health food stores and Asian groceries.

No amount of tea can compete with the benefits of an overall heart-healthy diet, however. Concentrate your cholesterol-cutting efforts on proven dietary strategies, such as reducing your intake of saturated fat and dietary cholesterol, advises Dr. Nicolosi.

Also, consume tea in moderation, especially if you're at risk for certain irregular heart rhythms, or arrhythmias. "Caffeine is a stimulant and has a tendency to accelerate the heart rate," says Connie Diekman, R.D., a dietitian in St. Louis and a spokesperson for the American Dietetic Association. People taking medication to control tachycardia, for example, may want to avoid caffeine.

See also Coffee Control

❧

TRIGLYCERIDE CONTROL

Taming the Forgotten Blood Fat

Don't have a clue as to what your triglyceride reading is—or even what triglycerides are? You should. There's evidence to suggest that elevated triglycerides may predict coronary heart disease, particularly in women and in people with diabetes.

WHAT'S YOUR LEVEL?

Like cholesterol, triglycerides are measured in milligrams/deciliter. Here are the National Cholesterol Education Program's guidelines for triglyceride levels.

200—Borderline high

400—High

1,000—Very high

Triglycerides, one of the major fats carried in blood, transport fatty acids that are derived from food or manufactured in the liver. Like cholesterol, triglycerides are measured in milligrams/deciliter.

In the famed Framingham Heart Study, which has tracked the health of the residents of Framingham, Massachusetts, for more than a generation, "a high triglyceride level (150 milligrams/deciliter or higher) appears to be an especially strong predictor of coronary heart disease in people who have low HDL cholesterol (less than 50 milligrams/deciliter)," says William P. Castelli, M.D., medical director of the Framingham Cardiovascular Institute, a wellness program at Metro West Medical Center.

What's more, "high triglycerides may play a more important role in women than in men," says Marla Mendelson, M.D., assistant professor of medicine at Northwestern University Medical School in Chicago. "Triglycerides are also higher in people with uncontrolled diabetes, which is itself a risk factor for heart disease."

Most experts agree that a high triglyceride reading should not be ignored, especially if it's coupled with high LDL cholesterol (the "bad" kind) and low HDL cholesterol (the "good" kind).

Conflicting Evidence

Triglycerides are essential to life. But consuming too many triglycerides can cause the body to make too much cholesterol. "There's an indirect relationship between high cholesterol and high triglycerides," says Frederic J. Pashkow, M.D., cardiologist at the Cleveland Clinic Foundation in Ohio and author of *50 Essential Things to Do When the*

SERVE UP SOME SALMON

Can the cholesterol-lowering omega-3 fatty acids in fatty fish such as salmon and albacore tuna help lower elevated triglycerides? According to some experts, the answer is yes.

"Studies have shown that these omega-3's can lower triglycerides as well as cholesterol," says James W. Anderson, M.D., professor of medicine and clinical nutrition at the University of Kentucky College of Medicine in Lexington and author of *Dr. Anderson's High-Fiber Fitness Plan.* "I recommend eating fish about twice a week. But you need to prepare the fish properly—broil or steam the fish rather than fry it."

Fish oil can help lower triglycerides as well, according to William P. Castelli, M.D., medical director of the Framingham Cardiovascular Institute, a wellness program at Metro West Medical Center in Massachusetts. Research conducted at Oregon Health Sciences University in Portland, says Dr. Castelli, showed that only fish oil lowered triglycerides to under 500 milligrams/deciliter in people whose triglycerides had topped 1,000 milligrams/deciliter. "As little as three to four grams of fish oil a day may be all that's needed," he says.

Doctor Says It's Heart Disease. "Triglycerides in the liver can be remetabolized and reconfigured as LDL cholesterol. The LDL formed as part of this triglyceride metabolism tend to be small and dense—the ones that are particularly atherogenic and dangerous."

Some studies have concluded that there is no direct association between triglyceride levels and cardiovascular risk, but other research has shown a significant association between the two. Here's a sampling of those studies.

In the Framingham Heart Study, high triglycerides in association with low HDL cholesterol were found to be an independent predictor of coronary heart disease in men and women over age 50. "People with high triglycerides and low HDL have many other problems that together greatly increase the risk of heart disease and diabetes," says Dr. Castelli. "These people can be missed in cholesterol screenings because their levels of total and LDL cholesterol aren't high."

Researchers in Norway analyzed triglyceride levels in 24,535 middle-aged women. The researchers found that as triglyceride readings increased, so did deaths related to coronary heart disease, as well as deaths from all causes. The researchers found no relationship between triglycerides and mortality in 25,058 men, however.

Researchers at Johns Hopkins University School of Medicine in Baltimore examined the relationship between cardiovascular disease and various blood fat measurements (total, HDL and LDL cholesterol and triglycerides) in about 1,400 women ages 50 to 69. Over a 14-year period, high triglycerides (over 200 milligrams/deciliter), particularly in combination with low HDL levels (under 50 milligrams/deciliter), were associated with an increased risk of death from heart disease. The researchers concluded that elevated triglycerides are an independent predictor of death from cardiovascular disease in women. Further, they recommended that "cholesterol screening guidelines should be re-evaluated to reflect the importance of HDL and triglyceride levels in determining risk in women."

Finally, people with high triglyceride levels may have more problems than others in lowering their LDL cholesterol, according to a study conducted at the Alton Ochsner Medical Foundation in New Orleans. Researchers followed the progress of 313 people enrolled in a rehabilitation program after having heart trouble. All of them had high cholesterol, and 39 had elevated triglycerides. The group was put on a low-fat, low-cholesterol diet for three months.

By the end of the study, the group as a whole had significant improvements in total, LDL and HDL cholesterol. But the people with high triglyceride levels had no significant improvement in LDL cholesterol or in the ratio of LDL to HDL. According to the researchers, people with high triglycerides may need more aggressive nondrug treatment to improve their cholesterol profiles.

Cutting These Fats Down to Size

"Ideally, your triglyceride level should be below 150 milligrams/deciliter," says Dr. Castelli. "People with coronary heart disease should probably have triglyceride levels below 100 milligrams/deciliter."

Most experts advise taking steps to lower high triglycerides, especially if you have low HDL cholesterol or high LDL cholesterol. "A high triglyceride level is a warning sign in many patients who have a predisposition for coronary heart disease," says Peter O. Kwiterovich

Heart-Healthy ♡
Indulgences

PEANUT BUTTER: IT'S NOT JUST FOR KIDS

Once a staple in children's lunchboxes and often a grownup favorite as well, peanut butter fell a bit out of favor a while ago when it was indicted as being too high in calories.

Surprise! Studies have now shown that peanut butter can aid in weight loss and cholesterol reduction. Peanut butter is rich in monounsaturated fats, which are considered beneficial to heart health. A study by Brigham and Women's Hospital and Harvard Medical School showed that dieters who ate large amounts of monounsaturated fats lost weight. And, thanks to the chemical structure of monounsaturated fats, peanut butter can also help lower levels of triglycerides and LDL cholesterol while maintaining HDL levels.

Other studies suggest additional benefits: sizeable drops in fibrinogen (a blood-clotting protein that's been linked to coronary artery disease when it's too high); glucose; insulin; and small, dense LDL particles. All of these factors can help to prevent a heart attack.

Here are some suggestions for incorporating peanut butter into your grownup diet.

- Spread a tablespoon on whole grain toast.
- In PB&J sandwiches, substitute fresh, sliced strawberries for jelly or jam.

Jr., M.D., professor of medicine and director of the Lipid Research and Atherosclerosis Unit at Johns Hopkins University School of Medicine in Baltimore and author of *The Johns Hopkins Complete Guide for Preventing and Reversing Heart Disease.* "It needs to be taken care of," he says.

Fortunately, say most doctors, you can usually lower a high triglyceride level with lifestyle changes. Here are some of the most common triglyceride-lowering strategies.

- Lose weight. "Triglycerides respond very well to weight reduction," says Dr. Kwiterovich. "Losing as little as five to ten pounds will significantly lower your triglycerides."

- Avoid alcohol. While studies have shown that a drink or two a day can help raise HDL cholesterol, alcohol can actually raise triglycerides by lowering the concentration of an enzyme used to break them down. "Even having a glass of wine with dinner every night can substantially raise triglycerides in people who are overweight or who have hereditary triglyceride problems," says Thomas Bersot, M.D., associate professor of medicine at the University of California, San Francisco.

- Avoid refined carbohydrates and sugars. Partially refined carbohydrates, including white flour and white rice; refined sugars such as those in candy; and even some high-sugar fruit juices such as orange juice will raise triglycerides in some people, says Dr. Castelli. "Switching to complex carbohydrates, such as whole wheat bread, brown rice, barley and rolled oats, can help lower triglycerides," he says.

- Exercise. "Walking just two miles a day can dramatically lower your triglycerides and raise your HDL cholesterol," says Dr. Castelli.

- Consider medication. If all else fails, your doctor may advise medication to help lower very high triglycerides, says Dr. Bersot. All drugs have potentially adverse effects, so discuss any possible downsides to the use of medication with your doctor, says Dr. Castelli.

VEGETABLES

More Than Just Side Dishes

For many of us, hating vegetables was as much a part of childhood as climbing trees or playing with dolls. Fortunately, most of us outgrew this disdain. As adults, we not only acquired a taste for beans, broccoli and bok choy, we began to appreciate their health benefits, too.

Vegetables are virtually fat-free, a boon if you're on a cholesterol-lowering program. "As you add more vegetables to your diet, you tend to consume less fat," says Martin Yadrick, R.D., a dietitian in Manhattan Beach, California, and a spokesperson for the American Dietetic Association. Vegetables are also loaded with fiber—both the insoluble kind, which promotes regularity and may lessen the risk of colon cancer, and the soluble variety, which helps trounce blood cholesterol levels. Soluble fiber is found in many of our favorite vegetables, including peas, corn and potatoes.

Best of all, veggies are so low in calories that you can eat virtually as many juicy beefsteak tomatoes, crisp snow peas and colorful red, orange and yellow peppers as you wish. "Americans like to eat lots of food," says Janet Lepke, R.D., a dietitian in Santa Monica, California, and a spokesperson for the American Dietetic Association. "When people eat less, they tend to feel deprived. But you can eat a lot of vegetables and feel good about it."

There's only one catch: You can cancel all of these benefits if you're in the habit of drowning your vegetables in butter, cream sauce or cheese sauce or loading them with salt. But you don't have to do without flavor. Using herbs, spices and condiments can transform a naked baked potato or plain green beans into veritable veggie delights. And your heart will thank you.

Greens, Glorious Greens

Some of the most compelling studies of the cholesterol-lowering benefits of vegetables (and fruits) were conducted in India. In one study, researchers put over 600 people who were at risk for coronary heart disease on a low-fat, low-cholesterol diet. Half of them were instructed to increase their intakes of fruits and vegetables to 400 or more grams (about five servings) a day; the others were not. After 12 weeks, the total cholesterol of the folks who ate the most fruits and vegetables dropped an average of 6.5 percent, and their "bad" LDL cholesterol dropped 7.3 percent. What's more, these folks' heart-healthy HDL cholesterol rose 5.6 percent. The total and LDL cholesterol of those who didn't eat the extra roughage remained the same.

In another Indian study, researchers put 400 people who had previously had heart attacks on a low-fat, low-cholesterol diet. As in the first study, half of these people were instructed to eat lots of fruits and

Heart-Healthy ♡
Indulgences

REAL SALAD DRESSING: OIL ISN'T ALL BAD

If you don't go overboard, dressings made with oil can have real benefits for your body and its engine, the heart.

Dressings made with canola or olive oil supply cholesterol-reducing monounsaturated fats, and those made with canola or walnut oil are good sources of alpha-linolenic acid, an omega-3 fatty acid. Omega-3's help your heart maintain its rhythm, and as a bonus, they may control the pain of rheumatoid arthritis and severe menstrual cramps and fight asthma, breast cancer and depression. Other vegetable oils provide phytochemicals such as beta-carotene, lutein and zeaxanthin, all of which fight cancer and protect your eyesight.

You have to use these oils in moderation, though, since they weigh in at 120 calories per tablespoon. If you drench your salad, the increased calories could offset any potential benefits.

Making your own salad dressing can be quicker than you think, not to mention that this one tastes good and is great for your heart.

RASPBERRY DRESSING

MAKES 1 CUP

    1   cup fresh or thawed and drained
        frozen raspberries
    ¼   cup balsamic vinegar
    4   teaspoons olive oil
        Pinch of ground black pepper

Place a fine sieve over a small bowl. Using the back of a spoon, press the raspberries through the sieve to remove the seeds. Add the vinegar, oil, and pepper to the puree and mix to combine.

PER 2 TABLESPOONS: 35 CALORIES, 2.3 G FAT (59% OF CALORIES), 0.1 G PROTEIN, 3.5 G CARBOHYDRATES, 0 MG CHOLESTEROL, 0.7 G DIETARY FIBER, 1 MG SODIUM vegetables; the other half were not. After three months, the total cholesterol of those who maxed out on fruits and vegetables plunged 27 points, from 226 to 199 milligrams/deciliter. Cholesterol readings in the control group fell, too, but less dramatically—14 points, from 229 to 215 milligrams/deciliter.

A Bumper Crop of Produce Pointers

You don't have to be a vegetarian to appreciate perfectly steamed asparagus or a fresh ear of corn. "There are lots of ways to enhance vegetables without using rich, fatty sauces," says Lisa Lauri, R.D., nutrition consultant at North Shore University Hospital in Manhasset, New York. These strategies can help maximize vegetables' nutrients—and flavors.

• Choose fresh or frozen vegetables over canned; they taste better and contain more nutrients. If you opt for frozen, read the package to make sure the product doesn't contain added salt or fat.

• Steam rather than boil vegetables, advises Los Angeles dietitian Bettye Nowlin, R.D., spokesperson for the American Dietetic Association. "Steamed vegetables are ready to eat in five minutes and retain most of their nutrients," she says. "They're nice and crunchy, too."

• Top baked potatoes and steamed vegetables with a blend of fat-free yogurt, garlic, a sprinkling of "light" salt and a dash each of curry and cayenne pepper. Delicious.

• Season vegetables with rice vinegar or another flavored vinegar, suggests Tammy Baker, R.D., a nutritionist in Cave Creek, Arizona, and a spokesperson for the American Dietetic Association. "You'll add flavor and avoid the butter dish," she says.

• Liven up cooked vegetables with herbs and spices, says Lauri. "Dill tastes wonderful on carrots," she says. You might also top a baked potato with chives, bring out the flavor of fresh green beans with garlic and rosemary or dust a sweet potato with ginger.

• At your next barbecue, pass up the ribs and grill up some vegetables. "Marinate sliced eggplant in low-sodium teriyaki sauce, ginger and garlic, then barbecue it," suggests Lepke. "It tastes delicious over rice." Try grilling big slices of mushrooms, peppers and zucchini, too. You can find suitable skewers or racks wherever grill accessories are sold, so food doesn't fall into the coals or burners.

• Want to make a low-fat cream sauce for vegetables? Blend a teaspoon each of low-fat margarine and flour, then heat for two minutes while slowly whisking in fat-free milk, suggests Marilyn Cerino, R.D., nutrition consultant at the Benjamin Franklin Center for Health of Pennsylvania Hospital in Philadelphia. Add seasonings appropriate to the vegetables.

• Prepare vegetables with flair, says Michael Klaper, M.D., health director of the Royal Atlantic Health Spa in Pompano Beach, Florida, and author of *Vegan Nutrition: Pure and Simple.* "You don't have to eat dry, plain vegetables. Have some fun with them. When you make pasta primavera, for example, use lots of green and yellow vegetables. Top rice or noodles with Chinese-style stir-fried vegetables. If you like East Indian cuisine, learn to make a vegetable curry."

• Don't shower vegetables with salt. A high-sodium diet may contribute to high blood pressure, which is no better for your heart than high cholesterol. "Cutting down on salt is like reducing the fat in your diet," says Neal Barnard, M.D., president of the Physicians Committee for Responsible Medicine in Washington, D.C. "You get used to it. So squirt a little lemon juice on your broccoli instead of salting it. It can make all the difference in the world."

VEGETARIAN DIET

The Right Way to Go Meatless

If the phrase "vegetarian diet" makes you think of alfalfa sprouts and tofu, it's time to update your thinking: Vegetarian cuisine is hot. Spurred in part by public recognition of its health benefits and by its new emphasis on elegance, ease of preparation and flavor, the meatless way of eating is surfing a renewed popularity unprecedented since the first wave of vegetarianism in the 1970s.

In fact, you may even consider yourself part of a new breed of vegetarian—the part-time vegetarian, who enjoys meatless meals prepared with pastas, grains and beans a few times a week.

In general, a vegetarian diet is low in fat and dietary cholesterol and high in fiber. In fact, a considerable amount of scientific evidence suggests that vegetarians are less likely to develop a number of chronic diseases, including coronary heart disease.

A vegetarian diet can provide your body with all of the nutrients that it needs, as long as you follow a few basic guidelines. Going vegetarian can also be delicious—and far easier than you might think.

Moving Away from Meat

Study after study suggests that vegetarianism and good heart health go hand in hand. Perhaps the best-known of these studies is the Lifestyle Heart Trial, led by Dean Ornish, M.D., president and director of the Preventive Medicine Research Institute in Sausalito, California, and author of *Dr. Dean Ornish's Program for Reversing Heart Disease.* In this study, Dr. Ornish and his colleagues placed 28 people with coronary atherosclerosis (fatty plaques in the arteries) on a low-fat vegetarian diet for a year. The diet derived about 10 percent of its calories from fat. To put this figure in perspective, the typical American diet gets about 37 percent of its calories from fat. These 28 people also quit smoking, engaged in moderate exercise, including walking, and performed stress management techniques such as meditation and yoga.

Another group of 20 people with arterial plaques were treated in the usual manner: Some took cholesterol-lowering drugs and all, on average, ate a diet deriving 30 percent of its calories from fat, a standard recommendation for people who want to lower their cholesterol.

After a year, researchers found that the arteries of 82 percent of the people who followed the low-fat vegetarian diet were less clogged than they had been before the study began. The drug-treatment group ended up with arteries that were more clogged. And—get this—the people whose arteries were the most closed to begin with showed the greatest improvement.

Researchers from the American Health Foundation in New York City compared the cholesterol levels of Seventh-Day Adventists who were vegans with those of people who ate the typical American diet. Vegans (pronounced VEE-gans), the strictest of all vegetarians, don't eat any foods from animal sources, including fish, poultry, dairy products and eggs. The researchers found that the Adventists' average total cholesterol was 25 percent lower and their average LDL cholesterol (the "bad" kind) was 38 percent lower.

In an 11-year study of over 1,900 vegetarians, researchers in Germany found that death from all causes was cut by one-half compared with the general population, while deaths from heart disease were reduced by one-third. Nondietary factors may have contributed to the vegetarians' longevity, said the researchers, who noted that most vegetarians are nonsmokers and are rarely overweight.

Researchers in China compared the cholesterol levels of 55 young Chinese Buddhist vegetarians with those of 59 Chinese medical students who ate both animal and vegetable substances. It was found that the vegetarians, who had been eating meatless diets for at least two years, consumed an average of 7 percent less fat, 3 percent less protein and 10 percent more carbohydrates than the students. Further, the students had significantly higher blood cholesterol levels—about 25 points higher in men and 36 points higher in women.

Ready for Veggies? Read This First

A vegetarian diet isn't automatically healthy. A steady diet of pizza, potato chips and chocolate cream pie may satisfy your taste buds, but not your body's need for vitamins and minerals. Here's how to make sure you get the nutrients you need without the fat and cholesterol you don't.

If you're on a vegetarian diet that allows dairy products, eat the low-fat or fat-free varieties. Whole milk cheese and whole milk are loaded with saturated fat, which can send your blood cholesterol skyward.

Also, when you dine out, make it clear that you want your food prepared with little or no fat. "A single serving of pasta primavera might contain four tablespoons of butter," explains Sue Chapman, executive chef at the Skylonda Fitness Retreat in Woodside, California.

Most important, make sure your diet contains adequate amounts of key nutrients. A vegetarian diet may fall short in protein, vitamin B_{12}, iron, zinc and calcium.

WHAT KIND OF VEGETARIAN ARE YOU?

There are several types of vegetarians, all of whom eat fruits, vegetables, grains and legumes. But some vegetarians eat dairy products and eggs, while others don't. Some people even qualify as part-time vegetarians, who eat meatless meals made with pastas, beans and grains several times a week. Here's a rundown of the most common types of vegetarians.

- Semivegetarians eat poultry, fish and dairy products.
- Lacto-ovo-vegetarians eat both dairy products and eggs.
- Lacto-vegetarians eat dairy products but not eggs.
- Ovo-vegetarians eat eggs but not dairy products.
- Vegans don't eat poultry, fish, dairy products or eggs.

"If you go on a vegetarian diet, you must educate yourself on how to get enough nutrients," says William P. Castelli, M.D., medical director of the Framingham Cardiovascular Institute, a wellness program at Metro West Medical Center in Massachusetts.

- If you omit all animal products from your diet, you may fall short in protein or vitamin B_{12}. So make sure your diet emphasizes protein-rich plant foods such as beans, peas and nuts.

Also, eat cereals fortified with vitamin B_{12} (a nutrient found naturally only in animal foods). If you give up only meat and not eggs or dairy foods, you'll be more likely to get the vitamin B_{12} you need, however.

- If you give up meat, you may also give up plenty of iron, zinc and calcium. You can get more of these vital nutrients by eating tofu, beans, peas and orange juice fortified with calcium.

See also Beans, Fiber, High-Fiber Cereals, Oats, Vegetables

WALKING

The Anywhere, Anytime Exercise

Walking is man's best medicine," said the Greek physician Hippocrates. If the good doctor were around today, he'd add that regular constitutionals can benefit women, too. In fact, walking is good medicine for virtually everyone, no matter what their age or level of fitness. Studies have shown that walking can help improve your cholesterol profile as well as lower blood pressure, reduce the risk of heart attack and stroke and control diabetes. "Walking may be the best medicine, because you can do it forever," says William P. Castelli, M.D., medical director of the Framingham Cardiovascular Institute, a wellness program at Metro West Medical Center in Massachusetts.

"It's thought that much of exercise's ability to reduce the risk of heart disease comes from its ability to increase HDL cholesterol," says James Rippe, M.D., director of the Center for Clinical and Lifestyle Research at Tufts University School of Medicine in Boston and coauthor of *Dr. James Rippe's Complete Book of Fitness Walking*. HDL cholesterol, the "good" kind, helps escort "bad" LDL cholesterol out of the body.

What's more, you don't need to own a closetful of expensive gear to reap the benefits of this simple yet effective exercise, say experts. "Walking is convenient and easy to do and requires no special equipment," says Darlene A. Sedlock, Ph.D., associate professor of kinesiology at Purdue University in West Lafayette, Indiana. "You can just step out your back door and go."

Step Lively to Stay Heart-Healthy

There's a significant amount of evidence to suggest that walking can promote heart health. Here are a few of those studies.

Investigators at the Institute for Aerobics Research in Dallas gave treadmill tests to more than 13,000 people and followed their fitness levels for eight years. They discovered that folks who walked for a half-hour a day had reduced levels of premature death nearly as impressive as those of people who ran 30 to 40 miles a week.

Researchers at Brigham Young University in Provo, Utah examined how walking affected the cholesterol levels of over 3,600 people. The ratios of total cholesterol to HDL cholesterol in folks who walked for 2½ to 4 or more hours per week were less likely to be elevated (a ratio of five or higher) than the ratios of those who didn't exercise regularly, according to Larry A. Tucker, Ph.D., professor and director of health promotion at Brigham Young.

Regular brisk walking increased HDL cholesterol in ten sedentary women who took part in a British study. These women (average age 47) followed a walking regimen for three months. Not only did brisk walking increase their HDL, but when researchers retested the women after six months of not walking, they discovered that the women's cardiovascular gains were lost.

Walking may also help stomp high levels of triglycerides (another blood fat implicated in heart disease) by stimulating an enzyme that carries triglycerides out of the blood, according to researchers at Baylor College of Medicine in Houston. These researchers had one group of 12 people take a single 2-hour walk. A second group didn't exercise at all. Then, 15 hours later, all of the participants ate a high-fat meal. After eating, the walkers' triglyceride readings were 31 percent lower than those of the nonexercisers.

How Fast? How Far?

You don't have to power-walk to prevent heart disease and promote health. Walking briskly for two miles every day, or nearly every day, is a great way to accumulate the half-hour of physical activity a day recommended by experts convened by the Centers for Disease Control and Prevention in Atlanta and the American College of Sports Medicine. What's more, when it comes to walking, speed doesn't determine effectiveness, say many experts.

Researchers at the Institute for Aerobics Research had 59 women walk three miles a day, five days a week, for six months. But each group walked at varying speeds. The first group of women walked a mile in 12 minutes. The second group walked a mile in 15 minutes. And the third group took 20 minutes to walk a mile. The fastest group of women had more impressive improvements in their overall fitness than the slowest group. But the HDL levels of all three groups jumped an average of 6 percent.

What about distance? Don't walk too far too fast, advises Ann Marie Miller, director of fitness and health services at the 92nd Street Y for Health, Fitness and Sport in New York City. "Walk a comfortable distance at a comfortable pace," she says.

Other experts agree. "You should be able to carry on a conversation while you walk," says exercise physiologist Peter Snell, Ph.D., assistant professor of internal medicine at the University of Texas Southwestern Medical Center at Dallas.

"If you can't talk without gasping for breath, slow down." Dr. Rippe concurs. "Give yourself time to make progress," he says.

The bottom line? Speed and distance are less important than consistency, say experts. "It's more important to walk at a comfortable pace on a regular basis," says Dan Rench, R.N., program director for cardiovascular rehabilitation at the Indiana Heart Institute at St. Vincent Hospital in Indianapolis. "If walking is fun, you'll probably stick with it."

Ready, Set, Walk!

Ready to hit the road? These expert tips can help you keep pace.

• Invest in a good pair of walking shoes. While you don't need hundred-dollar footwear, "you need more than ordinary tennis shoes for walking," says Dr. Rippe. The shoe you choose should be lightweight and padded at the heel and tongue as well as have an absorbent lining. Also, the shoe should bend easily across the ball of your foot and feature an uptilted sole to enhance your natural walking motion.

• Find a walking buddy, suggests Miller. Invite a coworker to take a "walk break" instead of a coffee break, then take a 15-minute stroll. You might even ask your spouse to share your walk before or after work.

• Walk with the weather in mind. In hot weather, wear loose-fitting, lightweight clothes, advises Dr. Rippe. And try to walk in the early morning or early evening, when the heat is less intense. Drink lots of water before and during your walk.

• In cold weather, dress in light layers that you can easily remove as your body warms up. "And watch your footing—your path could be icy and hazardous," says Miller. In truly stormy weather, climb up and down the stairs at home. *Caution:* If you have heart disease, diabetes, asthma or other health conditions, consult your doctor before walking in cold weather.

• Join a local walking club, suggests Miller. If you can't find one, consider starting your own.

• Forge new paths. Explore the grounds of a nearby botanical garden on foot. Or buy a book of local walking tours and hit the road.

• Imagine success. Visualize yourself on a brisk walk, feeling refreshed, positive and healthy. After all, a true power walk has just as much to do with the way you feel inside as with the speed of your stride.

See also Exercise

∽❦↢
_____

WALNUTS

Modern Benefits from an Ancient Food

In the early days of Rome, walnuts were considered a food fit for the gods and were named *Juglans regia* in honor of Jupiter. Not a bad endorsement. These days, however, we're more likely to bemoan the walnut's high content of fat and calories than to treat ourselves to this divinely delicious nut.

It's true that an ounce of walnuts contains about 180 calories and 17 grams of fat. But hold on: Eaten in moderation, walnuts may actually help lower your blood cholesterol without sabotaging your waistline.

How can the fat-laden walnut whittle down cholesterol? The answer lies in the type of fat this nut contains. Seventy percent of the fat in walnuts is polyunsaturated, which is gentler on your heart than the artery-plugging saturated fat found in red meat, cheese and butter. In fact, one study of the walnut notes that this nut's ratio of polyunsaturated to saturated fat is 7 to 1—"one of the highest among naturally occurring foods," the study states.

Walnuts are also rich in linolenic acid. This omega-3 fatty acid, also found in canola oil, is similar to the cholesterol-lowering omega-3's found in fatty fish.

A Nutty Way to a Healthier Heart

Two studies conducted at Loma Linda University in California indicate that walnuts can help put the crunch on elevated cholesterol levels.

Researchers first studied the lifestyles and diets of 31,208 Seventh-Day Adventists, searching for possible reasons why rates of heart disease and some cancers were lower in them than in other Americans. One of the researchers' findings: The Adventists who ate nuts (including peanuts and almonds as well as walnuts) five or more times a week were about half as likely to have a heart attack or to die from heart disease as those who ate nuts less than once a week.

And despite the fact that nuts are high in fat and calories, the most enthusiastic nut munchers in the study were not the heaviest. "The people who ate nuts five or more times a week were significantly thinner than those who didn't eat nuts at all," says Gary E. Fraser, M.D., Ph.D., professor of medicine at Loma Linda University School of Public Health. "These people ate nuts a small handful—about two ounces—at a time. They weren't sitting in front of the television with a can of nuts." In fact, being a couch potato is more likely to make you fat than eating certain foods, the study notes.

While this first study showed an association between nut consumption and heart health, it didn't prove a direct cause-and-effect relationship. So the Loma Linda researchers conducted a second study that examined the cholesterol-curbing effects of walnuts alone.

In this study, the researchers put 18 men with normal cholesterol on one of two low-fat diets. Half of the men followed a low-fat, low-cholesterol control diet. The second group of men ate the same diet but also consumed three ounces of walnuts a day (20 percent of calories from walnuts). At the midpoint of the two-month study, the men switched diets.

The men's total cholesterol averaged 182 milligrams/deciliter on the control diet but plunged to 160 milligrams/deciliter on the walnut diet. Further, the men's "bad" LDL cholesterol plummeted from 112 milligrams/deciliter on the control diet to 94 milligrams/deciliter on the walnut plan, a 16.3 percent drop. "This was a small study of 18 young men," says Dr. Fraser. "But we carefully controlled their diets and

LITTLE-KNOWN WALNUT HINTS

If you don't do much baking, you may not know much about how to shell, store or otherwise prepare walnuts, either. These simple hints can help.

- If you hate to crack walnuts, buy the preshelled kind. They're just as fresh and flavorful as the unshelled variety, says John Phillip Carroll, a chef in San Francisco and recipe author of *California the Beautiful Cookbook*.
- Refrigerate walnuts if you plan to use them within a few months, says Carroll. Otherwise, freeze the nuts. "Just wrap the walnuts well, so they won't absorb that freezer taste," advises Carroll.
- To get rid of walnuts' sometimes astringent aftertaste, which is caused by the tannin in the nuts' dry, papery skins, drop the nuts in boiling water for a minute or two (a process called blanching). Or simply add walnuts at the end of a recipe, says Carroll. "If the nuts sit in food for a while, their acidity may leach out," he says.

clearly documented that the walnut period was associated with a substantial decline in blood cholesterol."

The drops in cholesterol were mostly the work of walnuts' high content of polyunsaturated fat, says Dr. Fraser. But the reductions were "substantially larger than we would have predicted," he adds. "So it raises the question of some additional factor" in walnuts that may help deflate cholesterol levels, he says.

Grab a Handful of Heart Protection

The second Loma Linda study concluded that eaten in moderation, walnuts can be part of a cholesterol-lowering diet. But don't go overboard, says Mary Donkersloot, R.D., a dietitian in Beverly Hills, California, a spokesperson for the California Dietetic Association and author of *The Fast Food Diet*. "I'm hesitant to look at any food as a magic bullet," says Donkersloot. "It's one thing to add walnuts to a Waldorf salad, another to sit down and eat a bag of walnuts."

Translation: Eat walnuts in place of, not in addition to, other fats—especially saturated fats. Try these nutty serving suggestions.

• Sprinkle chopped shelled walnuts over steamed brussels sprouts or baked sweet potatoes.

• Toss a small amount of chopped walnuts into a salad. "The nuts will add flavor, texture and vitamin E," says Donkersloot.

• Add chopped walnuts to pancake batter, suggests John Phillip Carroll, a chef in San Francisco and recipe author of *California the Beautiful Cookbook.* Use about 1/4 cup of walnuts in a recipe that yields about eight three-inch pancakes. "You might also add 1/4 cup of mashed ripe banana and 1 1/2 cups of berries," suggests Carroll. To further reduce fat and cholesterol, prepare the batter with fat-free milk and egg substitute.

• If you have a food processor, make walnut sprinkles, suggests Carroll. These crispy fixings can add flavor and crunch to a variety of foods. Mix 1 cup of ground shelled walnuts with 1/2 cup of bread crumbs. Then bake at 325° for about 15 minutes, or until the sprinkles are crisp and golden brown. Stir in 1/4 teaspoon of cayenne pepper and one tablespoon of paprika, then cool. Use the sprinkles on salads, soups or pasta, in place of Parmesan cheese.

To make sweet, spicy sprinkles, replace the cayenne and paprika with two tablespoons of sugar and 1/2 teaspoon each of cinnamon and nutmeg. Stir these sprinkles into low-fat or fat-free yogurt, suggests Carroll.

~✣~

WEIGHT LOSS

Drop Pounds, Drop Cholesterol

Trying to scale down your cholesterol? Then chances are good that you're trying to scale down, period. "Being 20 to 30 percent over your ideal weight and having high cholesterol frequently go

---

EAT MORE AT HIGH NOON, LESS LATER ON

It's common knowledge that what we eat affects our weight. But so can when we eat it, according to Deepak Chopra, M.D., in his book *Perfect Weight*.

According to Ayurveda, the ancient Indian system of natural medicine, the body's "digestive fire" burns strongest at midday. Because digestion is stronger during this time, the body converts food into energy more efficiently, says Dr. Chopra. And in fact, many health professionals here in the West suggest eating a bigger breakfast and lunch and a lighter evening meal.

Make lunch your largest meal of the day and eat at approximately the same time each day, preferably between 12:00 and 12:30 P.M., suggests Dr. Chopra. "This one very simple change will make a profound difference in your metabolism," he says.

---

hand in hand," says John W. Zamarra, M.D., founding director of the Cardiac Rehabilitation Program at Placentia-Linda Community Hospital in Brea, California.

What's more, carrying excess pounds tends to deflate the body's level of "good" HDL cholesterol, which helps whisk the "bad" cholesterol, called LDL, out of the body. "People who are overweight generally have low HDL cholesterol, often accompanied by elevated total and LDL cholesterol," says Dr. Zamarra.

But chin up: Dropping those extra pounds can help you take control of your cholesterol. Further, shedding even a few pounds—5 to 10 percent of your initial weight—can significantly improve cholesterol levels, according to one study.

Love Handles? Check Your Cholesterol

Numerous studies have made a connection between body weight, elevated cholesterol levels and risk of coronary heart disease.

Using data from the second National Health and Nutrition Examination Survey, researchers from the University of Texas Health Science Center at Dallas Southwestern Medical School and other institutions examined the association between excess body weight and high blood cholesterol levels. These researchers conducted two separate studies: one with men, the other with women. Both reached the same conclusion: Excess body weight is associated with higher levels of total and LDL cholesterol and lower levels of HDL cholesterol in white men and women, whatever their ages.

Perimenopausal and menopausal women had lower HDL cholesterol and higher total and LDL cholesterol than premenopausal women, regardless of their weight. What's more, researchers discovered a stronger connection between body weight and triglyceride levels than between body weight and cholesterol. High levels of triglycerides (another type of blood fat that's implicated in heart disease) are now established as an independent risk factor for coronary heart disease in men and women, says William P. Castelli, M.D., medical director of the Framingham Cardiovascular Institute, a wellness program at Metro West Medical Center in Massachusetts.

Weigh In for the Last Time

Losing weight is one thing; keeping it off is quite another. But it can be done. These tips can help you shed those pounds permanently.

• Work that body. There's no way around it, experts say. "The only way to lose weight is to burn more calories than you consume—not just today or this week, but on a regular basis," says Leonard Doberne, M.D., an endocrinologist in Mount View, California.

More important, regular exercise can also maintain or even raise HDL cholesterol. While cutting back on dietary fat and cholesterol can often lower total blood cholesterol levels about 15 percent, it also tends to reduce HDL cholesterol, notes Dr. Doberne. "So the ratio of total cholesterol to HDL cholesterol, which appears to be of primary importance, is not always much improved," he says. "Exercise is the best way we know to raise HDL. That's why a weight-loss program aimed at improving the cholesterol ratio should include exercise."

• Avoid crash diets. They tend to slow the metabolism until the body kicks in to survival mode and starts storing fat like crazy, says Peg Jordan, R.N., in her book *How the New Food Labels Can Save Your Life*. Worse, once you start eating normally again, your metabolism is still sluggish, so any pounds you may have lost quickly return.

• Think twice about high-protein diets. People who once devoured pretzels and bagels—both laden with carbohydrates—have given them up in favor of high-protein foods like beef. These diets are all based on the incorrect notion that carbohydrates make you fat. When people lose weight on a hi-pro diet, they think it's because they're eating fewer carbohydrates, but it's really because they're eating fewer calories.

That said, high-protein diets vary in their approaches. Some, like the Atkins Induction diet, popularized in *Dr. Atkins' New Diet Revolution*, literally drip with artery-clogging saturated fat. And they lack the health-protective benefits of vegetables, fruits and whole grains. That in turn can lead to a jump in your cholesterol—and not the good HDL, either.

There are some moderate hi-pro diets, however, that have you cut back on starchy carbohydrates and sweets, substituting meat and tons of vegetables in their place. For most of us, that means swapping nutrient-empty white flour and sugar for nutrient-full protein and produce. So if you're going to go high-protein, better bets are Sugar Busters! and Dr. Barry Sears' The Zone, which focus on heart-healthy lean meat, poultry, fish and low-fat cheese, which are all low in saturated in fat.

• Cut the fat. Eating fatty foods such as processed lunchmeat, fried snacks and butter is the fastest route to weight gain, says Dr. Zamarra. "Fat contains nine calories per gram, more than twice as many as carbohydrates and protein, which have only four. You don't have to eat a lot of fatty foods to consume lots of calories."

• Eat more complex carbohydrates—whole grains, legumes, vegetables and fruits, recommends dietitian Deralee Scanlon, R.D., author of *Diets That Work*.

Why? Because the body expends more calories digesting and metabolizing complex carbohydrates. To transform 100 calories of carbohydrates into stored body fat, the body must use up 23 calories. But the body uses only 3 calories to convert 100 calories of dietary fat into body fat.

Foods high in complex carbohydrates also tend to be higher in fiber and lower in calories and fat. It's likely that these foods also are more filling and take longer to chew—two qualities that can help you reduce the amount you eat.

• Slow down. It takes about 20 minutes for your brain to let your body know that you've eaten enough, says Scanlon. If you eat quickly, you're likely to eat more than you really want.

If you rush through your meals like the Road Runner in the cartoon, Dr. Zamarra suggests that you try eating in a calm, settled atmosphere. A noisy, frenzied environment tends to make you eat faster—and more. Also, before you pick up your fork to begin eating, close your eyes and take a few deep breaths. "This can help you eat at a slower, more leisurely pace," he says.

See also Cooking, Exercise, Walking

WINE

Raise a Toast to Your Health

Imagine: You live in Paris, where the bread is fresh, the Brie is creamy, and the croissants are butter-soaked. Nevertheless, like other French men and women, your heart attack risk is less than half of the rate of your American *amis*.

Welcome to the French paradox.

This phrase refers to the mysterious fact that in some regions of France, people consume high-fat diets bursting with artery-clogging saturated fat and have high blood cholesterol, high blood pressure and smoking habits similar to those of Americans. Yet these folks have lower rates of coronary heart disease. Why do the French seem to get away with indulging in less-than-perfect health habits?

Many researchers believe that it may in part be the amount of wine the French consume. Studies here and abroad have found that people who consume moderate amounts of alcohol (even just one drink a day), as the French tend to do, have lower rates of coronary heart disease.

Experts aren't sure how wine may benefit the heart. But they do know that drinking wine (and other alcoholic beverages) in moderation tends to boost "good" HDL cholesterol. There's also evidence that alcohol increases the body's stores of a substance that helps keep the blood from clotting.

But questions remain. Some researchers question whether it's the alcohol or other substances in wine—such as antioxidants, the "supernutrients" such as vitamins C and E that have already been linked to reduced risk of heart disease and cancer—that exert the heart-healthy effects. And most experts agree: If you don't drink, don't start. Here's what is known about the relationship between wine and blood cholesterol.

Heart Protection in a Glass

Numerous studies have linked moderate alcohol intake with a low incidence of coronary heart disease.

French researchers examined the possible beneficial effects of red wine in a group of 56 healthy young men. Over a period of 14 days, the men drank, in random order, a little more than an ounce a day of three test beverages: red wine, an alternative form of alcohol, and alcohol-free red wine. Wine and alcohol both increased blood levels of HDL, but alcohol also increased triglycerides (another blood fat implicated in heart disease). There was no effect from alcohol-free red wine, other than decreasing HDL. The researchers concluded that a modest but noticeable beneficial effect was associated with moderate consumption of red wine compared with the other alcohol solution.

Some evidence suggests that wine consumption may help to explain why the French seem to be less vulnerable to a diet rich in saturated fat. Researchers in France analyzed data from 17 countries, including France. They concluded that the French population's high rate of wine consumption may offset their high intake of saturated fat. The researchers noted that people in Toulouse, France, consume about 38 grams of alcohol per day (34 grams of it as wine), compared with a much lower intake in Stanford, California. Further, the death rate from heart disease is 57 percent lower among men in Toulouse than among men in Stanford. But the researchers noted that alcohol "is a drug that, studies suggest, should be used regularly but only at moderate doses of about 20 to 30 grams per day." At this level of con-

WHAT'S BETTER FOR YOUR HEART, BEAUJOLAIS OR CHARDONNAY?

Which wine is better for the heart—red or white? It depends on whom you ask.

French researchers gave laboratory animals white wine, red wine or 6 percent ethanol. At first, all three groups showed about a 70 percent reduction in the clumping of blood platelets (which helps form blood clots). When the animals were deprived of alcohol for 18 hours, the platelet-clotting response increased 46 percent in the white-wine group and 124 percent in the ethanol group. But the animals that drank red wine showed a desirable 59 percent drop in clotting response.

"The platelets of the rats drinking red wine did not exhibit the rebound effect observed hours after alcohol drinking, eventually associated with sudden death and stroke in humans," wrote the researchers.

A study by researchers at the Kenneth L. Jordan Heart Foundation and Research Center in Montclair, New Jersey, on the other hand, found that white wine may be more beneficial.

The researchers had 20 men and women with high cholesterol consume 180 milliliters of either red or white wine every day for a month. Each group then switched to the other type of wine for another month. They ate whatever they wanted. While neither group had significant changes in total or "good" HDL cholesterol, the white wine lowered "bad" LDL cholesterol from 167 to 155 milligrams/deciliter. The researchers also found that people in both groups had a decreased blood-clotting response.

And investigators at the Kaiser Permanente Medical Care Program in Oakland, California, analyzed red-wine drinkers and white-wine drinkers and found that both groups have lower risks of coronary heart disease.

The upshot? "Classically, red wine has been thought to be more preventive than white wine, and there's some persuasive evidence in support of red wine—that it probably has a more complex effect within the body," says Frederic Pashkow, M.D., cardiologist at the Cleveland Clinic Foundation in Ohio and author of *50 Essential Things to Do When the Doctor Says It's Heart Disease*.

But not every expert agrees that red wine is a better cholesterol buster. "There's no difference (between red and white wine)," says William P. Castelli, M.D., medical director of the Framingham Cardiovascular Institute, a wellness program at Metro West Medical Center in Massachusetts. "All of the scientific evidence points to either one as helping to lower the risk of developing coronary heart disease."

sumption, the researchers said, "the risk of coronary heart disease can be decreased by as much as 40 percent."

Drinking wine and other alcoholic beverages may also boost levels of tissue-type plasminogen activator, or tPA. This substance, found naturally in the body, helps keep blood from clotting. In a study of over 600 men, those who reported drinking two or more drinks a day had 35 percent more tPA in their blood than men who said they rarely or never drank.

A study by researchers at Harvard University and Brigham and Women's Hospital in Boston examined the relationship between heart attack (myocardial infarction) and the type of alcoholic beverages consumed. Study participants who drank, on average, ½ to one drink a day or more of any alcoholic beverage—beer, wine or liquor—had a

Heart-Healthy ♡
Indulgences

FISH AND WINE: PAIRED FOR HEALTH

People who enjoy fish may optimize its heart-healthy benefits by having a glass or two of wine with their meal, especially if salmon or tuna is on the menu.

A study in Denmark suggests that this divine dinner duo can help prevent sudden cardiac death. The 291 men and women in the study were suspected of having ischemic heart disease, in which there is inadequate blood flow to the heart. The participants were asked about how much fish and wine they consumed, and the researchers measured the amount of heart-helping omega-3 fatty acids in their body fat.

The people with higher levels of omega-3's had higher heart rate variability (HRV) than those with low levels. Simply put, low HRV is a significant indicator of sudden cardiac death in people with ischemic heart disease, so eating fish may decrease the risk of an unexpected fatal heart attack. (Oily fish like salmon and tuna have more generous amounts of omega-3's than pale, lean fish like haddock or flounder.)

The researchers also noted that people who ate a lot of fish often tended to drink more wine. While wine may have some positive health effects of its own, it seems that consuming wine and fish together can maximize your health benefits.

lower risk of heart attack than nondrinkers. Levels of HDL were significantly higher in all beverage categories in drinkers than in nondrinkers. The researchers credited the protective effect of alcohol, in large part, to the increased HDL. They suggested that regular consumption of small to moderate amounts of alcoholic beverages, regardless of the type, reduces the risk of myocardial infarction and further suggested that there is benefit from increases in HDL levels.

Can Wine "Rustproof" Your Arteries?

Some researchers theorize that it's the antioxidants in wine, not the alcohol, that cause the beneficial effect. Some studies have shown that red wine has a potent antioxidative capacity and has reduced the oxidation of "bad" LDL cholesterol in test-tube studies. (Oxidation is a chemical process that appears to increase the likelihood of LDL cholesterol collecting in the arteries.)

"Red wine contains antioxidants," says Peter O. Kwiterovich Jr., M.D., professor of medicine and director of the Lipid Research and Atherosclerosis Unit at Johns Hopkins University School of Medicine in Baltimore and author of *The Johns Hopkins Complete Guide for Preventing and Reversing Heart Disease*. (White wine also contains antioxidants.)

These antioxidant compounds may hinder the buildup of fatty deposits in the coronary arteries, says John D. Folts, Ph.D., director of the University of Wisconsin Coronary Artery Thrombosis Research and Prevention Lab at the University of Wisconsin Hospital and Clinics in Madison.

One compound that has gotten a lot of attention is resveratrol, a fungus-fighting compound found in the skin of grapes. Animal studies have shown that purified resveratrol appears to lower cholesterol, and one study has theorized that resveratrol may be the active ingredient in wines that reduces blood cholesterol.

Researchers at the University of California, Davis, drew blood samples from a group of people with normal cholesterol levels. After removing the LDL cholesterol from the samples, the researchers mixed the LDL with phenolic compounds drawn from red wine. They found that the phenolic compounds reduced the oxidation of LDL cholesterol by 60 to 98 percent.

A separate study at Queen Elizabeth Hospital in Birmingham,

England, provided the first evidence that red wine seems to enhance antioxidant activity in the blood. Researchers had ten people consume two lunches over two days. At one of the lunches, each person drank a glass of red wine. At the other, they drank no wine. A half-hour after each meal, each volunteer gave the first of several blood samples taken over a four–hour period.

After the wine meal, the antioxidant levels in the people's blood rose, reaching a peak after 90 minutes. More significantly, their antioxidant levels were higher than those shown to inhibit oxidation of LDL cholesterol in test-tube experiments. After the wine-free meal, the blood showed little change in antioxidant activity.

Before You Imbibe

A bottle of Bordeaux won't work magic on clogged arteries, says William P. Castelli, M.D., medical director of the Framingham Cardiovascular Institute, a wellness program at Metro West Medical Center in Massachusetts. And some experts feel that wine shouldn't be touted as a cholesterol buster at all. One study concluded that "the protective effects of alcohol come at the cost of life-shortening alcohol abuse by large numbers of people." And other studies note that while a moderate amount of alcohol may have a protective effect, risk increases with the amount consumed.

The bottom line? If you don't drink, don't start, says Frederic Pashkow, M.D., cardiologist at the Cleveland Clinic Foundation in Ohio and author of *50 Essential Things to Do When the Doctor Says It's Heart Disease.* "There are other ways besides drinking to improve your cholesterol profile, including reducing the fat in your diet and getting regular exercise," says Dr. Pashkow. "Nevertheless, if you're already having a drink a day, and your doctor says it's okay, then it's fine to continue to drink in moderation."

See also Alcohol, Grape Juice

YOGA

The Great Stress Reducer

If the word *yoga* makes you think of turbaned East Indian yogis or spaced-out hippies chanting in incense-clouded rooms, take a new look at this centuries-old discipline. In recent years, yoga has cast off its counterculture image and gone mainstream.

More and more Americans are embracing yoga, a form of active meditation that originated in India 4,000 years ago, to banish back pain, relieve arthritis and increase their strength and flexibility. Others use yoga as a natural tranquilizer to help soothe emotional stress. "Practicing yoga can help you enter what some people call inner state, in which the mind becomes more tranquil," says Michael Lee, director of Phoenix Rising Yoga Therapy in Housatonic, Massachusetts. Westerners are most familiar with hatha yoga, which focuses on breathing and on assuming a series of poses, or *asanas.*

And if you think you have to twist yourself into a pretzel to reap the physical and mental benefits of yoga, think again. "Yoga postures can be very uncomplicated," says Christine Kaur, a yoga instructor in Los Angeles who has taught the discipline for over 20 years. "But even the simplest postures can produce tremendous health benefits." And one of these benefits may be a decrease in cholesterol levels, suggests F. J. Chandra, D.P.H., in the *Journal of the International Association of Yoga Therapists.*

The Link to Cholesterol

While there's not much in the way of scientific proof that yoga can help curb cholesterol, there is evidence that stress can elevate cholesterol and may even damage the coronary arteries, setting the stage for heart disease. Yoga has been shown to temporarily alter automatic bodily functions such as heartbeat and breathing. According to research led by Herbert Benson, M.D., chief of the Division of Behav-

ioral Medicine at Beth Israel Deaconess Medical Center in Boston, associate professor of medicine at Harvard Medical School and author
of *The Relaxation Response*, yoga can slow the heart rate, bring
oxygen consumption and the breathing rate below resting levels and
even reduce blood pressure in some people.

More directly, some studies have shown that stress management
techniques such as yoga can reduce cholesterol levels, according to
Dean Ornish, M.D., president and director of the Preventive Medicine
Research Institute in Sausalito, California. Dr. Ornish includes the practice of yoga techniques, including breathing, meditation, visualization
and progressive relaxation, in his program for people with heart disease. "The use of cholesterol-lowering drugs, while often helpful, is
based on the presumption that cholesterol is the primary determinant
of atherosclerosis," says Dr. Ornish, author of *Dr. Dean Ornish's Program for Reversing Heart Disease*. But Dr. Ornish says he has become
increasingly convinced that other psychological factors, including
emotional stress, can contribute to the development of heart disease.

And at least one study, while small, seems to support the theory
that yoga can help deflate elevated cholesterol. Researchers in India
had six healthy young men practice yoga breathing exercises each
day. At the end of six months, their total serum lipids (blood fats such
as cholesterol and triglycerides) reportedly fell dramatically.

Do-It-Yourself Techniques

Interested in exploring the benefits of yoga for yourself? Consider
enrolling in a yoga class, suggests Lee. To find a class, check the
yellow pages under "Yoga Instruction" or see if your local YM/YWCA
offers yoga instruction. Before you sign up for a class, though, make
sure the instructor emphasizes yoga as a form of relaxation rather than
as a form of spiritual enlightenment or rigorous exercise. Lee suggests
sitting in on a class or two, so you can see the class—and the instructor—in action.

"Find an instructor you feel compatible with," suggests Lee. "Avoid
instructors who believe that yoga has to 'hurt to work' or who are very
results-oriented and believe that you have to reach a certain level of
achievement." Finding the right yoga class is like trying on clothing—
you have to find what fits.

In the meantime, try these simple stress-relieving postures. Lee suggests the following exercise.

1. While standing or sitting, place your arms behind your back and clasp your hands. If your hands don't meet comfortably, "cheat" by holding the ends of a towel.
2. Stretch upward and outward. Feel the stretch across your chest (but don't stretch so far that it hurts).
3. Take a deep breath. As you exhale, continue to stretch, opening up your chest and keeping your hands clasped.
4. Continue to take full, deep breaths, drawing air down into your belly and letting it out again. After several minutes, take one more breath and slowly unclasp your hands.

Kaur suggests this simple breathing exercise.

1. Sit comfortably in a chair or couch. Keep your spine fairly straight and your shoulders back and relaxed.
2. With your eyes closed, close off your right nostril with your right thumb and take 26 long, deep breaths through your left nostril. Then close off your left nostril with your left thumb and repeat the process, breathing through your right nostril. Let yourself become completely calm and try to enter a peaceful, focused state.

See also Stress Management

YOGURT

A Versatile Treat That Does Double Duty

Strictly speaking, yogurt can't lower blood cholesterol. But this custardlike concoction can help turn the tide on high-flying cholesterol levels. That's because low-fat yogurt (rather than the whole milk variety) contains three grams or less of fat per cup, while the fat-free variety doesn't have a speck of fat. And as you'll see, there are lots of uses for "skinny" yogurt: The fruit-flavored kind makes a tasty snack, dessert or topping, while the plain variety stands in for high-fat ingredients in everything from dips to desserts.

And what is good for your cholesterol level is good for your bones, too. An excellent source of calcium, yogurt can help battle osteoporosis, the bone-thinning disease that preys on people later in life. One cup of low-fat or fat-free yogurt contains more calcium than a glass of milk and meets roughly one-third to one-half of your Daily Value for calcium (1,000 milligrams). What's more, yogurt contains very little lactose, a milk sugar that leaves some people unable to drink milk or eat other calcium-rich dairy products. So yogurt is a good source of calcium for these lactose-intolerant folks. Yogurt is brimming with protein and B vitamins, too.

Not all yogurt fits into a cholesterol-conscious diet, however. Avoid varieties that contain whole milk and sugar. Some brands of yogurt contain up to 350 calories and 11 grams of fat.

Dips, Desserts and More

Whether you're craving a savory dip or a succulent dessert, yogurt can help fit the bill—deliciously. Try these suggestions.

• Top pancakes and waffles with low-fat or fat-free fruit-flavored yogurt instead of butter and syrup.

• For a tasty breakfast treat, stir a few tablespoons of wheat germ or high-fiber cereal into a cup of fat-free vanilla yogurt.

• To make a deliciously different dressing for chicken salad, blend vanilla low-fat or fat-free yogurt with fat-free mayonnaise, suggests Marilyn Cerino, R.D., nutrition consultant at the Benjamin Franklin Center for Health of Pennsylvania Hospital in Philadelphia.

• Create a creamy dip for raw vegetables or other low-fat snacks by mixing fat-free yogurt with fat-free sour cream, dill and garlic, says Janet Lepke, R.D., a dietitian in Santa Monica, California, and a spokesperson for the American Dietetic Association.

• Substitute fat-free plain yogurt for sour cream or buttermilk in homemade baked goods. "Drain the yogurt through a piece of cheesecloth or a coffee filter," suggests Cerino. "You'll end up with a nice, thick product that you can add to muffins and quick breads."

• Jazz up plain or vanilla yogurt with some chopped fresh fruit, suggests Lisa Lauri, R.D., nutrition consultant at North Shore University Hospital in Manhasset, New York.

• Whip up a frothy yogurt "smoothie" by blending fat-free plain or vanilla yogurt with fresh fruit or juice.

• If you're an ice cream maven, enjoy low-fat or fat-free frozen yogurt rather than premium ice cream, suggests William P. Castelli, M.D., medical director of the Framingham Cardiovascular Institute, a wellness program at Metro West Medical Center in Massachusetts. You'll save yourself 30 or more grams of fat. It's possible to have too much of a good thing, however, and low-fat treats are no exception. "Some people eat twice as much frozen yogurt as ice cream and end up gaining weight," says Dr. Castelli. "So be aware of how much you're eating."

Most people with diabetes can eat foods that contain artificial sweeteners, says Lauri. But if you are pregnant and have diabetes (gestational diabetes), she recommends that you avoid products flavored with these substances just to be on the safe side. "Choose plain yogurt and mix in some fruit," suggests Lauri.

THE BREAKTHROUGH MENU PLAN

Cut Cholesterol 30 Points in 30 Days

Want to gorge on three squares (plus snacks) a day and lower your cholesterol 30 points in 30 days? Have we got a meal plan for you!

This nutritionist-approved menu plan, designed to lower cholesterol 30 points in 30 days, provides about 2,000 calories a day, with 55 percent of calories from complex carbohydrates (starches), 20 percent from fat, 15 percent from protein and 10 percent from simple carbohydrates (sugars). And of the 20 percent of calories from fat, only about 5 percent come from saturated fat. The typical U.S. diet contains 13 percent of calories from saturated fat.

As for cholesterol, this plan includes 150 milligrams a day, which is half of the American Heart Association's recommended limit of 300 milligrams a day. The plan also contains more fiber and less sodium than the typical U.S. diet. All meals provide one serving.

To reduce your cholesterol 30 points in 30 days, you have to switch from the typical American diet (which gets about 37 percent of its calories from fat) to the diet outlined in the following pages—and follow it to the letter. If you eat 30 percent of calories from fat, for example, your cholesterol may drop about 15 points in 30 days.

But if you think lowering your cholesterol while enjoying tasty, filling meals sounds too good to be true, you're in for a pleasant surprise. Sharon Faelten, senior editor of *Prevention* Women's Health Books, followed this very diet, with amazing results.

Before she went on the diet, a cholesterol test showed that her total cholesterol was 238 milligrams/deciliter—borderline high, according to laboratory standards. After following this menu plan for the suggested 30 days, she took a follow-up test and found that her cholesterol had dropped 28 points, to 210 milligrams/deciliter.

More important, the food tasted great, and there was plenty of it—three meals a day (including pizza, pasta and tacos) plus two snacks (from devil's food cookies to hot, chewy bake-and-eat pretzels).

"The first night, I made the haddock, rice and broccoli for dinner. My husband, a meat-and-potatoes kind of guy, said, 'Very good, Sharon. Very good.' The compliments kept coming. On Day 3, I made the chicken breast with sautéed cabbage. 'This stuff is good, Sharon,' he remarked. On Day 6: 'This is really, really good!'

"The combination of salsa and yogurt in the chicken fajitas is surprisingly good," says Faelten. "It's surprising, too, how far just a little oil goes.

"I tried new foods that I discovered I like better than standard fare," she says. "The veggie burger (lunch, Day 3) is quite tasty and light—much easier on the digestion than a beef burger.

"I was delighted that my cholesterol went down, and I had no trouble continuing the diet after the follow-up test. As a bonus, I found I had more energy than ever. After staying up past 1:00 A.M. on a Friday, I had enough energy to get up before 7:00 A.M. to go hiking. Then I went home and started painting the bedroom."

It's a diet anyone can follow.

Menu plan: Anita Hirsch, R.D., former nutritionist, Rodale Test Kitchen.

Menu plan review: Sonja L. Connor, R.D., research associate professor of clinical nutrition at the Oregon Health Sciences University in Portland.

Day 1

Breakfast

¾ cup grape juice
1 cup oatmeal with ¼ cup raisins and ¼ cup fat-free milk
⅛ wedge cantaloupe

Lunch

1 cup cooked pasta with ½ cup low-sodium marinara sauce
Tossed salad: 1 cup chopped romaine lettuce, ½ cup shredded carrots
  and ½ cup shredded red cabbage, dressed with 2 teaspoons canola
  oil, 2 tablespoons vinegar and a dash of sweet basil
Garlic bread: 2 slices toasted Italian bread, brushed with 2 teaspoons
  olive oil and rubbed with 1 clove fresh garlic

Dinner

Fresh vegetable platter: ¼ cup cauliflower, ¼ green pepper, sliced,
  and ¼ cup chopped mushrooms
Vegetable dip: ¼ cup fat-free yogurt, flavored with 1 scallion, chopped
3 ounces broiled haddock
¾ cup steamed rice
1 cup steamed broccoli with ¼ teaspoon fresh ginger or a dash of
  dried ginger
½ cup cubed winter squash and ¼ cup crushed pineapple, sprinkled
  with nutmeg

Snacks

2 ounces fat-free unsalted pretzels
1 apple, sliced and topped with ½ cup low-fat vanilla yogurt,
  2 teaspoons wheat germ and 1 tablespoon slivered almonds

DAILY TOTALS: 1,932 CALORIES, 34 G TOTAL FAT, 3.6 G SATURATED FAT, 65 MG CHOLESTEROL,
30 G DIETARY FIBER, 1,457 MG SODIUM

Day 2

Breakfast

½ English muffin with 1 tablespoon strawberry spread and 1 teaspoon diet margarine

½ cup low-fat vanilla yogurt with 2 tablespoons wheat germ

1 orange

Lunch

1 cup grape juice

Turkey sandwich: 1 ounce white meat turkey on 2 slices whole wheat bread with lettuce, tomato and 1 teaspoon mustard

Tossed salad: 3 cups chopped greens, 1 carrot, sliced, and ¼ cup chickpeas, dressed with 2 teaspoons olive oil and 2 tablespoons flavored vinegar

4 graham crackers

Dinner

1 cup low-sodium minestrone soup

3 ounces lean roast beef

1 baked potato, topped with butter-flavored sprinkles and a dash of garlic powder

½ cup steamed brussels sprouts, topped with 1 tablespoon vinegar and a dash of dry mustard

2 slices Italian bread with 2 teaspoons diet margarine

1 cup canned peaches, in juice

Snacks

½ bagel with 1 tablespoon low-fat cream cheese

1 pear

DAILY TOTALS: 1,982 CALORIES, 36 G TOTAL FAT, 9 G SATURATED FAT, 96 MG CHOLESTEROL, 38 G DIETARY FIBER, 1,796 MG SODIUM

Day 3

Breakfast

¾ cup orange juice
1 cup ready-to-eat raisin bran cereal with ½ cup fat-free milk
2 dried figs

Lunch

Vegetable burger on whole wheat bun with lettuce, tomato, onion
and mustard
½ cup commercially prepared three-bean salad
1 carrot and 1 stalk celery, cut into sticks
½ cup low-fat coffee-flavored yogurt
1 tangerine or other fresh fruit

Dinner

Tossed salad: 3 cups chopped romaine lettuce, 2 slices tomato,
½ carrot, sliced, 2 radishes and 2 slices cucumber, dressed with
2 teaspoons olive oil and 2 tablespoons vinegar
3 ounces grilled or baked chicken breast, rubbed with fresh garlic and
½ teaspoon olive oil
1 cup steamed brown rice
Savory cabbage: ½ cup shredded cabbage and ¼ cup chopped
onions, sautéed in 2 teaspoons olive oil, ½ teaspoon savory and
½ teaspoon dill
1 baked apple with 2 tablespoons maple syrup

Snacks

3 fat-free devil's food cookies
2 cups air-popped popcorn with ½ teaspoon butter-flavored sprinkles

DAILY TOTALS: 1,969 CALORIES, 38 G TOTAL FAT, 8.6 G SATURATED FAT, 95 MG CHOLESTEROL,
39 G DIETARY FIBER, 1,909 MG SODIUM

Day 4

Breakfast

1½ cups ready-to-eat multigrain cereal with ½ cup fat-free milk,
    sprinkled with 5 almonds, chopped
½ red grapefruit

Lunch

1 cup low-sodium split pea soup
1 toasted English muffin with 2 teaspoons diet margarine
¾ cup low-fat or fat-free strawberry yogurt with 1 teaspoon rice bran
    or wheat germ

Dinner

Pork stir-fry: 1 ounce lean pork loin, 1 cup sliced bok choy, ½ cup
    snow peas, ¼ cup diced red peppers and ¼ cup diced celery,
    stir-fried in 1 teaspoon minced fresh garlic, 2 teaspoons canola oil
    and a dash of sesame oil
1½ cups steamed brown rice with a dash of poultry seasoning or sage
Tossed salad: 1 cup shredded romaine lettuce, ¼ cup chopped red
    onions and 2 radishes, dressed with 1 tablespoon lemon juice and
    2 teaspoons olive oil
1 banana or other fresh fruit

Snacks

1 cup grapes
1 bake-and-eat soft pretzel (2½ ounces, baked without salt)

DAILY TOTALS: 1,941 CALORIES, 40 G TOTAL FAT, 6.8 G SATURATED FAT, 33 MG CHOLESTEROL,
25 G DIETARY FIBER, 1,465 MG SODIUM

Day 5

Breakfast

1 English muffin with 2 teaspoons diet margarine

Breakfast blender drink: 1 cup fat-free milk and ½ cup fresh or unsweetened frozen strawberries, blended until frothy

Lunch

Pita sandwich: 1 ounce cubed low-fat Cheddar cheese, ½ cup chopped spinach, tomato and onion, stuffed in a pita and dressed with 2 tablespoons fat-free dressing (your choice)

1 carrot and 1 stalk celery, cut into sticks

1 cup low-fat yogurt (your choice)

Dinner

2 slices pizza (ask for only half the cheese)

Tossed salad: 3 cups chopped greens, ¼ cup broccoli, ¼ cup chickpeas, ¼ tomato, sliced, and 1 tablespoon chopped onions, dressed with 2 tablespoons fat-free dressing (your choice)

1 cup grapes

Snacks

2 cups cooked pasta with ½ cup low-sodium marinara sauce

2 unsalted pretzels (2 ounces)

1 banana

DAILY TOTALS: 1,899 CALORIES, 28 G TOTAL FAT, 7 G SATURATED FAT, 50 MG CHOLESTEROL, 26 G DIETARY FIBER, 2,473 MG SODIUM

Day 6

Breakfast

³/₄ cup orange juice

Egg substitute, scrambled with 1 tablespoon fat-free milk in a nonstick pan

1 potato, sliced and sautéed with 1 tablespoon diet margarine, 2 tablespoons chopped onions and ¹/₂ clove fresh garlic, minced, in a nonstick pan

2 slices toasted whole wheat bread with 2 teaspoons fruit spread

Lunch

1 cup low-sodium lentil soup

Tossed salad: 3 cups chopped greens, ¹/₂ cup sliced carrots and ¹/₄ cup sliced onions, dressed with 2 teaspoons olive oil and 1 tablespoon vinegar

1 toasted English muffin

Dinner

Chicken fajita: 3 ounces chicken strips (prepared in a low-fat manner), ¹/₄ cup mashed avocado, ¹/₄ cup salsa, ¹/₄ cup fat-free plain yogurt, 1¹/₂ teaspoons olive oil, 1 teaspoon lime juice and 1 teaspoon fresh cilantro in 1 flour tortilla

1¹/₂ cups steamed brown rice, flavored with 2 tablespoons salsa and ¹/₈ teaspoon chopped jalapeño peppers

10 low-fat tortilla chips (1 ounce)

Snacks

1 cup fresh or canned chunked pineapple, in juice

1 carrot, cut into sticks, with ¹/₄ cup commercially prepared fat-free herbed yogurt cheese

DAILY TOTALS: 1,902 CALORIES, 45 G TOTAL FAT, 7.3 G SATURATED FAT, 77 MG CHOLESTEROL, 29 G DIETARY FIBER, 1,717 MG SODIUM

Day 7

Breakfast

½ bagel with 1 tablespoon light cream cheese
1 cup low-fat vanilla yogurt with 2 teaspoons wheat germ
½ mango, cubed

Lunch

2 ounces scallops, ½ cup chopped mushrooms, ¼ cup sliced onions,
¼ cup chopped celery and ¼ cup chopped green peppers,
sautéed in 1 teaspoon sesame oil, 1 tablespoon low-sodium soy
sauce, 1 clove fresh garlic, minced, and 1 teaspoon grated fresh
ginger
2 cups steamed rice
1 fortune cookie

Dinner

2 cups low-sodium vegetable soup
Tossed salad: 1 ounce flaked water-packed tuna, 4 cups chopped
romaine lettuce, ¼ cup shredded carrots and 1 radish, dressed with
1 teaspoon olive oil and 1 tablespoon vinegar
Baked pita crisps: 1 pita, brushed with 2 teaspoons olive oil and
assorted herbs and spices, broiled and broken into pieces
1 cup fresh fruit (grapes, apples and oranges)

Snacks

2 graham crackers with 1 tablespoon peanut butter and 1 cup fat-free
milk
1 banana

DAILY TOTALS: 2,030 CALORIES, 40 G TOTAL FAT, 10 G SATURATED FAT, 61 MG CHOLESTEROL,
25 G DIETARY FIBER, 1,761 MG SODIUM

Day 8

Breakfast

¾ cup orange juice

1 cup oatmeal with ¼ cup raisins and ½ cup fat-free milk

1 slice toasted whole wheat bread with 1 teaspoon diet margarine
and 1 tablespoon apple butter

Lunch

1 cup low-sodium tomato soup

¼ to ½ cup commercially prepared three-bean salad (add ¼ cup
chopped red onions, basil and 2 tablespoons red wine vinegar)

2 slices rye bread with 2 teaspoons diet margarine

1 peach, nectarine or other fresh fruit

Dinner

Bulgur salad: 1 cup cooked bulgur, 2 tablespoons parsley, ½ tomato,
chopped, and 1 teaspoon lemon juice

Broiled skinless chicken breast

1 potato, baked, with 2 tablespoons fat-free sour cream and
2 teaspoons diet margarine

1 cup chopped spinach, sautéed in 1 teaspoon olive oil, ¼ cup
chopped onions and 1 clove fresh garlic, minced

1 hard roll (2 ounces) with 1 tablespoon diet margarine

2 cups cubed watermelon or other fruit

Snacks

2 cups air-popped popcorn with butter-flavored sprinkles and
1 teaspoon Parmesan cheese

1 fresh fig

DAILY TOTALS: 1,968 CALORIES, 41 G TOTAL FAT, 7 G SATURATED FAT, 84 MG CHOLESTEROL,
41 G DIETARY FIBER, 1,850 MG SODIUM

Day 9

Breakfast

¾ cup ready-to-eat fortified oat cereal with ½ cup fat-free milk
1 sliced banana

Lunch

1 oat bran and raisin muffin (2 ounces)
1 cup low-fat yogurt (your choice)
1 orange, sliced

Dinner

1 cup low-sodium vegetable soup (add ¼ cup white beans and 1 clove fresh garlic, minced, if desired)
3 ounces baked flounder
¼ cup chopped cabbage, sautéed in 2 teaspoons canola oil and ground red pepper (to taste) and served over 1 cup steamed rice
1 slice cornbread with 2 teaspoons diet margarine
1 baked apple with ½ teaspoon cinnamon and 2 teaspoons brown sugar

Snacks

6 graham crackers with 1 tablespoon almond butter or peanut butter
½ cup fat-free milk

DAILY TOTALS: 1,748 CALORIES, 33 G TOTAL FAT, 4 G SATURATED FAT, 68 MG CHOLESTEROL, 31 G DIETARY FIBER, 1,273 MG SODIUM

Day 10

Breakfast

1 cup cooked oat bran cereal with 1 tablespoon rice bran or wheat germ
2 cups cubed honeydew, casaba or other melon

Lunch

1 applesauce muffin (1 ounce) with 2 teaspoons diet margarine
½ cup 2% cottage cheese with 2 cups fresh fruit (your choice)

Dinner

1 cup low-sodium vegetable juice
1 cup low-sodium green pea soup
Spinach salad: 2 cups spinach, ¼ cup sliced mushrooms, ¼ cup chopped red onions and 1 clove fresh garlic, minced, dressed with 2 teaspoons olive oil and 2 tablespoons vinegar
4 garlic breadsticks (4 ounces)

Snacks

2 fig bars
1 orange
Fresh vegetable plate: 1 cup carrot sticks and ½ cup broccoli florets
Vegetable dip: 2 tablespoons commercially prepared fat-free herbed yogurt cheese

---

DAILY TOTALS: 1,796 CALORIES, 41 G TOTAL FAT, 11 G SATURATED FAT, 10 MG CHOLESTEROL, 44 G DIETARY FIBER, 1,985 MG SODIUM

Day 11

Breakfast

1 cup hot cereal with 1 tablespoon wheat germ and 2 tablespoons maple syrup

Fruit compote: 2 tablespoons prunes, 2 tablespoons figs and 2 tablespoons raisins, cooked in 2 tablespoons orange juice and 2 tablespoons water

Lunch

1 cup low-sodium turkey vegetable soup

Tossed salad: 4 cups chopped romaine lettuce, dressed with 2 teaspoons olive oil and 2 tablespoons vinegar

2 slices toasted whole wheat bread

1 cup low-fat yogurt (your choice)

Dinner

3 ounces pork medallions in tomato sauce, served over 1 cup egg noodles

1½ cups steamed green beans and chopped carrots

2 slices rye bread with 2 teaspoons diet margarine

Streusel apple: 1 apple, baked with 1 tablespoon low-fat flavored yogurt, ½ tablespoon oats and 1 teaspoon brown sugar

Snack

2 ounces low-sodium pretzel chips with mustard

DAILY TOTALS: 1,996 CALORIES, 41 G TOTAL FAT, 7.2 G SATURATED FAT, 122 MG CHOLESTEROL, 32 G DIETARY FIBER, 1,721 MG SODIUM

Day 12

Breakfast

1 cup ready-to-eat bran cereal with ½ cup fat-free milk
2 slices toasted whole wheat bread with 2 teaspoons diet margarine
1 banana

Lunch

½ grapefruit
Pasta salad: 1 cup cooked pasta, 1 ounce water-packed tuna, ½ cup
   snow peas, ½ cup frozen or canned plain artichoke hearts and
   2 scallions, chopped, dressed with 1 tablespoon low-fat mayonnaise,
   1 tablespoon vinegar, fresh basil and parsley
1 slice pumpernickel bread with 2 teaspoons diet margarine

Dinner

Chicken kabobs: 2 ounces cooked cubed chicken breast with ¼ pepper,
   chunked, ½ tomato, chunked, 5 mushrooms, chunked, and ⅓ onion,
   chunked, marinated in 2 teaspoons olive oil, 2 teaspoons lemon juice,
   2 teaspoons low-sodium soy sauce, 1 tablespoon chopped parsley,
   1 clove fresh garlic, minced, ¼ chili pepper, minced, and ¼ teaspoon
   red-pepper flakes
1½ cups steamed brown and wild rice, tossed with thyme or parsley
1 frozen fruit bar

Snacks

1 cup grapes
1 oat bran and raisin muffin (2 ounces)

DAILY TOTALS: 1,895 CALORIES, 33 G TOTAL FAT, 5 G SATURATED FAT, 65 MG CHOLESTEROL,
38 G DIETARY FIBER, 2,065 MG SODIUM

Day 13

Breakfast

Four 4-inch buckwheat pancakes with 4 tablespoons maple syrup
Citrus salad: ¼ cup grapefruit sections and ½ cup orange sections

Lunch

Egg drop soup: 1 cup hot low-fat chicken stock with 2 tablespoons
    egg substitute
Chicken teriyaki with vegetables (low-fat, low-calorie frozen entrée)
1½ cups steamed brown rice with chives
Wonton chips: 3 wonton wrappers, misted with nonstick cooking spray
    and baked
3 kumquats or ½ cup fresh or canned chunked pineapple, in juice

Dinner

Omelette: ⅓ cup chopped mushrooms and ⅓ cup chopped onions,
    sautéed in 2 teaspoons olive oil and folded into ½ cup beaten egg
    substitute
2 slices toasted whole wheat bread with 2 teaspoons diet margarine
    and 1 tablespoon strawberry spread
1 apple, sliced, with 1 tablespoon natural peanut butter

Snacks

1 carrot, cut into sticks
2 slices melba toast with 1-ounce chunk low-fat Swiss cheese

DAILY TOTALS: 1,805 CALORIES, 42 G TOTAL FAT, 11.4 G SATURATED FAT, 123 MG CHOLESTEROL,
32 G DIETARY FIBER, 1,978 MG SODIUM

Day 14

Breakfast

³/₄ cup tropical fruit juice

2 whole grain waffles, topped with ½ cup low-fat yogurt (your choice) and ½ cup blueberries

Lunch

Turkey sandwich: 1 ounce low-fat turkey breast lunchmeat and 1 ounce low-fat Swiss cheese on 2 slices rye bread with lettuce, tomato and 2 teaspoons mustard

1 carrot, cut into sticks

Curry dip: ¼ cup fat-free plain yogurt and ¼ cup fat-free mayonnaise, blended with ½ teaspoon curry and 1 clove fresh garlic, minced

Dinner

3 ounces boneless, skinless chicken breast, poached with ¼ cup chopped onions, ¼ cup chopped carrots and 1 tablespoon parsley and served over 1 cup steamed chopped spinach

Hawaiian rice: 1 cup cooked brown rice with ½ cup snow peas, 4 pieces baby corn and ¼ cup water chestnuts, sautéed in 1 teaspoon peanut oil and ¼ teaspoon ground red pepper and tossed with ¼ cup drained chunked pineapple

1 sweet potato, baked or steamed (top with cinnamon, if desired)

½ mango, sprinkled with ¼ cup macadamia nuts

Snack

1 slice cocoa angel food cake (¹/₁₂ cake) with ½ cup fresh raspberries

---

DAILY TOTALS: 2,108 CALORIES, 53 G TOTAL FAT, 11 G SATURATED FAT, 101 MG CHOLESTEROL, 37 G DIETARY FIBER, 2,228 MG SODIUM

Day 15

Breakfast

1 peach bran muffin (2 ounces)
1 cup fat-free milk
1 pear

Lunch

1 cup low-sodium vegetable soup (add ¼ cup diced carrots and ¼ cup chopped kale, if desired)
Tossed salad: 2 cups chopped greens, 2 tablespoons chopped cabbage and ¼ cup diced celery, dressed with ¼ cup fat-free yogurt blended with 1 clove fresh garlic, minced
2 slices whole wheat bread with 1 tablespoon natural peanut butter
1 cup grapes

Dinner

2 ounces sliced lean roast beef
Mushroom barley: ⅓ cup chopped mushrooms, sautéed in 2 teaspoons olive oil and ¼ teaspoon thyme and added to 1 cup cooked barley
1 cup steamed sliced carrots
1 slice Italian bread with 1 teaspoon diet margarine
½ cup peaches with ½ cup pureed strawberry sauce

Snacks

1 bake-and-eat soft pretzel (2½ ounces, baked without salt)
1 apple, sliced and sprinkled with cinnamon

DAILY TOTALS: 1,895 CALORIES, 40 G TOTAL FAT, 9 G SATURATED FAT, 108 MG CHOLESTEROL, 49 G DIETARY FIBER, 1,666 MG SODIUM

Day 16

Breakfast

1 English muffin with 2 teaspoons diet margarine, 1 tablespoon fruit spread and 1 teaspoon wheat germ

1 orange

Lunch

1 potato, baked, with chives and 2 tablespoons fat-free sour cream

Spinach salad: 2 cups chopped spinach, ½ carrot, chopped, ¼ cup chopped mushrooms and ¼ cup chopped onions, dressed with 2 tablespoons low-fat dressing (your choice)

2 slices Italian bread with 1 tablespoon diet margarine

Dinner

3 ounces grilled snapper

½ cup black beans with 4 tablespoons tomato salsa, served over 1 cup steamed rice

1 cup zucchini, sautéed in 2 teaspoons olive oil with ¼ cup chopped onions and 1 clove fresh garlic, minced

½ cup fresh blueberries and ¼ cup fat-free vanilla yogurt

Snacks

2 oatmeal cookies (1 ounce each) with 1 cup fat-free milk

2 cups cubed watermelon

DAILY TOTALS: 1,809 CALORIES, 34 G TOTAL FAT, 5.5 G SATURATED FAT, 39 MG CHOLESTEROL, 30 G DIETARY FIBER, 1,823 MG SODIUM

Day 17

Breakfast

¾ cup orange juice

1 cup cooked bulgur with ¼ cup apricot nectar, 1 tablespoon chopped dried fruit bits, ¼ cup fat-free milk and 2 teaspoons oat bran

Lunch

1 cup low-sodium vegetable soup

Roast beef sandwich: 1 ounce sliced lean roast beef on a hard roll (2 ounces) with romaine lettuce, onion and 2 teaspoons mustard

Fresh veggie plate: 1 cup cauliflower florets, 1 carrot, cut into sticks, and 2 or 3 cherry tomatoes

2 tablespoons fat-free dressing (your choice)

Dinner

Cheese and spinach lasagna (low-fat frozen entrée)

1 cup steamed broccoli with ¼ teaspoon basil

Garlic bread: 2 slices toasted Italian bread, brushed with 2 teaspoons olive oil and rubbed with 1 clove fresh garlic

Fruit plate: 1 kiwifruit, sliced, and 3 strawberries, sliced

2 reduced-fat cookies

Snacks

2 cups air-popped popcorn with ¼ teaspoon of your choice of seasonings: curry powder, Worcestershire sauce, Parmesan cheese, dill or butter-flavored sprinkles

1 peach or other seasonal fruit

DAILY TOTALS: 1,726 CALORIES, 34 G TOTAL FAT, 6.7 G SATURATED FAT, 27 MG CHOLESTEROL, 32 G DIETARY FIBER, 2,212 MG SODIUM

Day 18

Breakfast

¾ cup grape juice
1 large shredded-wheat biscuit with ½ cup fat-free milk
1 oat bran and blueberry muffin

Lunch

1 cup low-sodium Manhattan clam chowder
1 slice toasted whole wheat bread, topped with 1 ounce low-fat,
   low-sodium Cheddar cheese, ¼ cup sliced onions and 1 slice tomato
   and broiled
Tossed salad: 2 cups chopped greens, ¼ cup chopped mushrooms and
   ¼ cup shredded carrots, dressed with 2 tablespoons low-fat dressing
   (your choice)
½ cup fresh pineapple wedges

Dinner

2-ounce chicken burger patty on a bun (1 ounce) with lettuce, tomato
   and onion
Oven fries: 1 potato, thinly sliced and baked with garlic powder, Italian
   seasoning or other spices
1 cup canned or homemade baked beans, without salt
½ cup applesauce with a dash of cinnamon

Snacks

½ cup low-fat frozen yogurt (your choice)
1 bake-and-eat soft pretzel (2½ ounces, baked without salt)
3 vanilla wafers

DAILY TOTALS: 1,939 CALORIES, 29 G TOTAL FAT, 8.5 G SATURATED FAT, 103 MG CHOLESTEROL,
46 G DIETARY FIBER, 2,203 MG SODIUM

Day 19

Breakfast

1 cup cooked oatmeal with 2 teaspoons rice bran and ½ cup fat-free milk

1 orange

Lunch

Tacos: 1 ounce extra-lean ground beef, 8 tablespoons cooked lentils, 3 tablespoons stewed tomatoes, ¼ tomato, chopped, ½ cup chopped lettuce, ½ ounce shredded low-sodium, low-fat Cheddar cheese, 2 tablespoons mashed avocado and 2 tablespoons fat-free sour cream, layered in 2 taco shells

1 cup steamed rice (add 2 tablespoons salsa, if desired)

Dinner

Beef stew: 2 ounces lean beef (bottom round), simmered in 1 cup water with 1 cup chunked carrots, 1 cup chunked potatoes, ½ cup sliced onions, 1 clove fresh garlic, minced, 2 tablespoons parsley, 1 teaspoon basil and 1 teaspoon savory

1 cup cooked barley or barley/rice mix, flavored with ¼ teaspoon marjoram, ¼ teaspoon chopped onions and ¼ teaspoon garlic powder

1 slice whole wheat bread or low-sodium cornbread with 2 teaspoons diet margarine

Snacks

1 apple

2 ounces unsalted pretzels

2 cups air-popped popcorn with butter-flavored sprinkles

DAILY TOTALS: 1,870 CALORIES, 31 G TOTAL FAT, 8 G SATURATED FAT, 84 MG CHOLESTEROL, 40 G DIETARY FIBER, 737 MG SODIUM

Day 20

Breakfast

1 toasted bagel with 2 tablespoons fat-free cream cheese
1 baked apple with 1 teaspoon diet margarine and 1 tablespoon maple syrup

Lunch

Tossed salad: 2 cups chopped greens with ¼ cup shredded carrots, ¼ cup diced celery, ¼ cup shredded cabbage, ¼ cup frozen or canned plain artichoke hearts and 1 tablespoon ground chile pepper (if desired), dressed with 2 tablespoons fat-free dressing (your choice)
6 whole wheat crackers
1 cup fresh strawberries or other seasonal fruit

Dinner

Greek salad: 4 cups chopped romaine lettuce, 1 ounce feta cheese, ¼ cup sliced mushrooms, ¼ cup chickpeas and 2 olives, dressed with 2 tablespoons lemon juice and 1 tablespoon olive oil
3 ounces haddock fillet
1 potato, chunked and roasted with 1 teaspoon rosemary
Ratatouille: ¼ cup tomato sauce, ½ cup chopped eggplant, ¼ tomato, chopped, ½ zucchini, sliced, and ¼ cup chopped celery, served over ½ cup cooked orzo
¼ cup hummus, spread over 1 pita bread
½ cup rice pudding with raisins

Snacks

2 fresh or dried figs
½ cup fat-free yogurt (your choice)
1 orange

DAILY TOTALS: 1,940 CALORIES, 44 G TOTAL FAT, 8.5 G SATURATED FAT, 81 MG CHOLESTEROL, 42 G DIETARY FIBER, 2,486 MG SODIUM

Day 21

Breakfast

1 cup oatmeal with ½ cup sliced strawberries, 1 tablespoon brown sugar and ½ cup fat-free milk

2 slices toasted whole wheat bread with 2 teaspoons diet margarine

Lunch

Pizza: ¼ ready-made pizza crust, ¼ cup tomato sauce, 1 ounce reduced-fat mozzarella cheese, ¼ cup roasted red peppers, ½ teaspoon olive oil, ½ teaspoon hot-pepper flakes, ¼ cup chopped green peppers, ¼ cup chopped red peppers, ¼ cup cooked white beans and ¼ cup chopped spinach

1 carrot, cut into sticks

½ cup grapes

Dinner

3 ounces lamb (loin chop)

Potato sauté: 1 potato, sliced, ¼ cup chopped mushrooms, ¼ cup chopped onions, 1 tablespoon parsley and 1 clove fresh garlic, minced, sautéed in ½ cup chicken stock

1 cup steamed brussels sprouts, seasoned with herbes de provence, savory or lemon juice

1 roll (2 ounces) with 2 teaspoons diet margarine

1 poached peach, sliced, with nutmeg and cinnamon

Snacks

2 slices toasted cinnamon raisin bread

4 fig bars

DAILY TOTALS: 1,881 CALORIES, 39 G TOTAL FAT, 10 G SATURATED FAT, 98 MG CHOLESTEROL, 29 G DIETARY FIBER, 2,012 MG SODIUM

Day 22

Breakfast

¾ cup orange juice
1 cup ready-to-eat oat cereal with ½ cup fat-free milk
1 banana, sliced

Lunch

1 cup chicken chow mein (low-calorie frozen entrée)
2 cups steamed white rice
1 fortune cookie or fresh fruit

Dinner

3 ounces baked orange roughy
1 cup barley, topped with ½ cup chopped mushrooms and ¼ cup
    sliced onions sautéed in 2 teaspoons olive oil and ½ cup tomato
    salsa
1 cup steamed cauliflower

Snacks

1 whole grain waffle, topped with ½ cup frozen yogurt (your choice)
    and 2 tablespoons chocolate syrup
1 peach, sliced

DAILY TOTALS: 1,868 CALORIES, 23 G TOTAL FAT, 6 G SATURATED FAT, 66 MG CHOLESTEROL, 27 G DIETARY FIBER, 1,589 MG SODIUM

Day 23

Breakfast

1 bagel, topped with 2 tablespoons fat-free cream cheese mixed with
1 tablespoon chopped dates
1 orange

Lunch

Salmon salad: 2 ounces canned red salmon, arranged on 2 cups
chopped romaine lettuce with 1 green onion, thinly sliced, and
¼ cup chopped mushrooms and dressed with 2 teaspoons olive oil
and 2 tablespoons vinegar
Cucumber and onion salad, dressed with ¼ cup fat-free plain yogurt
and dill
Garlic bread: 2 slices toasted Italian bread, brushed with 2 teaspoons
olive oil and rubbed with 1 clove fresh garlic

Dinner

1 cup light cheese tortellini
½ cup tomato sauce
½ cup steamed green beans, flavored with ⅛ teaspoon olive oil, fresh
rosemary, grated lemon rind and butter-flavored sprinkles
3 soft breadsticks (1½ ounces total) with 2 teaspoons diet margarine
Mini fruit salad: ½ cup sliced apples and ¼ cup grapes, drizzled with
½ cup low-fat vanilla yogurt

Snacks

Pronto pinto dip: ½ cup cooked pinto beans, mashed, with
2 tablespoons chunky salsa and 2 tablespoons fat-free sour cream
22 baked tortilla chips

DAILY TOTALS: 1,785 CALORIES, 42 G TOTAL FAT, 8.3 G SATURATED FAT, 86 MG CHOLESTEROL,
25 G DIETARY FIBER, 2,496 MG SODIUM

Day 24

Breakfast

1 cup oatmeal with 1 tablespoon brown sugar and ½ cup fat-free milk
1 tangerine or other seasonal fruit

Lunch

1 cup low-sodium black bean soup
1 cup polenta with 1 cup stewed tomatoes (with onions) and
    ⅛ teaspoon ground chili pepper
½ cup grapes

Dinner

Tossed salad: 2 cups chopped romaine lettuce, ¼ cup frozen or
    canned plain artichoke hearts and ¼ sweet red pepper, chopped,
    dressed with 2 teaspoons olive oil and 2 tablespoons vinegar
3 ounces roasted skinless chicken breast
Three-grain pilaf: ⅓ cup steamed rice, ⅓ cup steamed barley and
    ⅓ cup steamed buckwheat, tossed with ¼ cup diced onions, ¼ cup
    diced celery and ¼ cup diced mushrooms sautéed in chicken stock,
    ¼ teaspoon dried tarragon, ¼ teaspoon rosemary and ¼ teaspoon
    dry mustard
1 cup steamed sliced carrots and beets, dressed with 2 teaspoons olive
    oil, 2 teaspoons vinegar and ½ teaspoon basil

Snack

2 rye crackers with 1 ounce low-fat mozzarella cheese

DAILY TOTALS: 2,201 CALORIES, 38 G TOTAL FAT, 8.9 G SATURATED FAT, 78 MG CHOLESTEROL,
22 G DIETARY FIBER, 1,485 MG SODIUM

Day 25

Breakfast

1 slice toasted whole wheat bread with 2 teaspoons diet margarine
½ cup fat-free vanilla yogurt with 2 chopped dried figs and
2 teaspoons wheat germ

Lunch

Chef's salad: 2 cups chopped mixed greens (romaine lettuce and
spinach) with 1 ounce shredded fat-free Swiss cheese, 1 ounce
julienne roasted turkey (without skin), ¼ cup sliced cucumbers,
¼ cup sliced radishes, ½ cup shredded carrots and 3 or 4 cherry
tomatoes, dressed with 2 tablespoons fat-free dressing (your choice)
3 breadsticks (1¼ ounces each)
1 cup unsweetened applesauce with cinnamon

Dinner

3 ounces broiled salmon
1½ cups white and wild rice with 2 teaspoons slivered almonds,
1 tablespoon sautéed diced onions, 2 teaspoons chopped parsley
and a pinch of saffron
1 artichoke, dressed with 1 tablespoon lemon juice, 1 teaspoon olive
oil, 1 tablespoon fat-free Parmesan cheese and butter-flavored
sprinkles
¼ wedge cantaloupe

Snack

Tropical shake: ½ cup fat-free milk, ½ cup orange juice, 1 banana and
5 strawberries, whipped until thick and frothy

DAILY TOTALS: 1,734 CALORIES, 32 G TOTAL FAT, 6.9 G SATURATED FAT, 80 MG CHOLESTEROL,
34 G DIETARY FIBER, 2,089 MG SODIUM

Day 26

Breakfast

¾ cup ready-to-eat raisin bran cereal with ½ cup fat-free milk
1 peach

Lunch

1½ cups low-sodium turkey noodle soup
1 sweet potato, baked with 1 tablespoon maple syrup, cinnamon and
    nutmeg
Spinach salad: 1 cup chopped spinach, ½ cup shredded carrots, ¼ cup
    alfalfa sprouts and ¼ cup sliced onions, dressed with 2 teaspoons
    olive oil and 2 tablespoons vinegar
1 pumpernickel roll (1 ounce) with 1 teaspoon diet margarine
Mixed fruit: ½ cup canned unsweetened pears, ¼ cup sliced apples,
    ¼ cup grapes, 1 dried fig, 2 tablespoons raisins

Dinner

Vegetable lasagna (low-fat, low-calorie frozen entrée)
½ cup steamed sliced carrots with a dash of fresh or dried ginger
Garlic bread: 2 slices toasted Italian bread, brushed with 2 teaspoons
    olive oil and rubbed with 1 clove fresh garlic
1 lemon sorbet bar

Snacks

Tropical delight: ½ cup orange juice, 1 banana, sliced, and 1 tablespoon
    slivered almonds, whipped until frothy
2 popcorn rice cakes

DAILY TOTALS: 1,874 CALORIES, 39 G TOTAL FAT, 4.7 G SATURATED FAT, 29 MG CHOLESTEROL,
32 G DIETARY FIBER, 2,215 MG SODIUM

Day 27

Breakfast

Two 4-inch whole grain pancakes

Scrambled eggs: ¼ cup egg substitute, scrambled with 1 tablespoon fat-free milk in a nonstick pan

1 ounce turkey sausage

Lunch

Rice jambalaya: 1½ cups cooked rice with ¼ cup cooked diced ham, ¼ cup cooked cubed chicken breast, ¼ cup crushed tomatoes, ¼ cup diced celery, ¼ cup chopped onions, ¼ cup chopped green peppers and ¼ cup chopped mushrooms

2 buttermilk biscuits (¾ ounce each)

Fruit compote: 1 orange, sectioned, and 1 kiwifruit, sliced

Dinner

Stuffed potato: 1 baked potato with 2 ounces low-fat Cheddar cheese, ½ cup steamed broccoli, ¼ cup chopped onions and 1 clove fresh garlic, minced

1 carrot, cut into sticks, with 1 tablespoon fat-free blue cheese dressing

½ cup fat-free pudding, made with fat-free milk

Snacks

1 bake-and-eat soft pretzel (2½ ounces, baked without salt)

1 stewed apple, topped with ¼ cup fat-free vanilla yogurt and drizzled with honey

---

DAILY TOTALS: 1,727 CALORIES, 26 G TOTAL FAT, 11 G SATURATED FAT, 147 MG CHOLESTEROL, 24 G DIETARY FIBER, 2,401 MG SODIUM

Day 28

Breakfast

1 toasted bagel with 2 tablespoons fat-free cream cheese and
1 tablespoon strawberry spread
1 cup vanilla fat-free yogurt
½ cup mixed berries

Lunch

3 ounces London broil (top round), marinated in ¼ teaspoon
Worcestershire sauce, garlic and herbs and grilled
2 ears grilled corn on the cob with butter-flavored sprinkles
Veggie kabobs: ½ cup chunked mushrooms, ½ cup chunked onions
and ½ cup chunked peppers, grilled on skewers and brushed with
fat-free dressing (your choice)
2 breadsticks
2 cups cubed watermelon

Dinner

Pita pizza: 1 pita, smothered with ¼ cup tomato puree, 2 ounces
shredded fat-free or reduced-fat mozzarella cheese, ⅓ cup sliced
mushrooms, 1 clove fresh garlic, minced, and ¼ cup chopped
onions
Tossed salad: 3 cups chopped greens, dressed with 2 tablespoons
vinegar and 2 teaspoons olive oil
1 frozen fruit bar

Snack

2 cups air-popped popcorn with butter-flavored sprinkles

DAILY TOTALS: 1,735 CALORIES, 38 G TOTAL FAT, 14 G SATURATED FAT, 121 MG CHOLESTEROL,
29 G DIETARY FIBER, 1,707 MG SODIUM

Day 29

Breakfast

1 cup ready-to-eat oat cereal with almonds, topped with 1 banana, sliced, and ½ cup fat-free milk

½ grapefruit

Lunch

1 cup low-sodium chicken noodle soup

Ham and cheese sandwich: 1 ounce low-fat ham and 1 ounce low-fat American cheese on a hard roll (1 ounce) with lettuce, tomato and mustard

1 carrot and 1 stalk celery, cut into sticks

Flavored sparkling water

Dinner

Turkey tenders: 3 ounces white-meat turkey, sautéed with 2 teaspoons olive oil, ½ cup chopped kale, ¼ cup sliced mushrooms, ¼ cup chopped onions, ¼ cup sliced bell peppers and ¼ cup chopped hot peppers and served over 1 baked potato

Pasta salad: 1 cup cooked macaroni, ¼ cup chopped zucchini, ¼ cup chopped onions and ¼ cup frozen or canned plain artichoke hearts, dressed with 2 tablespoons low-fat mayonnaise and sprinkled with basil and pepper

2 slices whole wheat bread with 2 teaspoons diet margarine

Snacks

1 apple

½ cup fat-free vanilla yogurt with 1 tablespoon chopped walnut topping

1 bake-and-eat soft pretzel (2½ ounces, baked without salt)

DAILY TOTALS: 1,959 CALORIES, 42 G TOTAL FAT, 5 G SATURATED FAT, 57 MG CHOLESTEROL, 28 G DIETARY FIBER, 2,020 MG SODIUM

Day 30

Breakfast

2 slices toasted raisin bread with ½ cup reduced-fat ricotta cheese
1 banana

Lunch

1 cup low-sodium vegetarian chili, served over 1½ cups steamed rice
Carrot and raisin salad: ¼ cup shredded carrots and ¼ cup raisins,
    served on ½ cup chopped romaine lettuce with 2 tablespoons walnuts
    and dressed with 2 tablespoons fat-free yogurt and 1 tablespoon light
    mayonnaise
½ cup low-fat yogurt (your choice) with ½ cup raspberries

Dinner

1 cup pasta
Red clam sauce: ¼ cup low-sodium stewed tomatoes, ¼ cup
    low-sodium tomato sauce, ¼ cup shredded carrots and 1½ ounces
    rinsed and chopped canned clams
1 slice Italian bread
2 almond biscotti or 1 fat-free cookie (your choice)

Snacks

4 small gingersnap cookies (1 ounce total)
1 pear

DAILY TOTALS: 2,103 CALORIES, 37 G TOTAL FAT, 10.5 G SATURATED FAT, 76 MG CHOLESTEROL,
28 G DIETARY FIBER, 1,182 MG SODIUM

500-FOOD FAT AND CHOLESTEROL COUNTER

Choose Foods That Work in Your Favor

Put away your calculator: The chart that begins on page 246 can make it simpler than you may think to stick to a cholesterol-lowering diet. The best part? No number crunching is necessary (unless you want to do it, of course).

Like most other fat and cholesterol counters, this chart divvies up food into categories, from beans to vegetables. In between, you'll find breakfast foods, desserts, snack foods, fish and shellfish, meats and so forth. But this chart is designed a bit differently from those you may have used in the past. The difference? It ranks foods by the amount of saturated fat per serving—"low," "acceptable" or "high"—rather than by the amount of dietary cholesterol. Most experts agree that saturated fat is the healthy heart's worst enemy. The more you stick to foods in the "low" category—and there's a delicious array to choose from—the less saturated fat you'll eat and the healthier your diet will be.

As long as your overall calorie and cholesterol intake is reasonable, that is. As odd as it may seem, some foods contain a low percentage of saturated fat but pack lots of calories and cholesterol. For example, a couple of slices of frozen French toast drizzled with low-calorie syrup will "cost" you less than two grams of saturated fat, but they provide significant calories and cholesterol. Another example: Both three ounces of tofu and a fast-food ham-and-cheese breakfast croissant get 54 percent of their calories from fat. But compare the calories, cholesterol and saturated fat content, and it's easy to see why breakfast croissants should be an occasional indulgence.

Here's some other information that you'll need to use this chart.

• We've rounded calorie and cholesterol counts to the nearest whole number and fat and saturated fat values to the nearest tenth of a gram.

FOOD	PORTION	CALORIES
BEANS, BEAN PRODUCTS AND OTHER LEGUMES		
LOW		
Adzuki beans, boiled	½ cup	147
Baked beans with pork, canned	½ cup	134
Black beans, boiled	½ cup	114
Broad beans (fava beans), boiled	½ cup	94
Chickpeas, canned	½ cup	143
Green peas, boiled	½ cup	67
Lentils, boiled	½ cup	114
Lima beans, boiled	½ cup	108
Refried beans, canned	½ cup	135
Snap beans (green beans), boiled	½ cup	22
Soybeans, boiled	½ cup	149
Soybean sprouts, raw	½ cup	45
Split peas, boiled	½ cup	116
Three-bean salad, canned	⅓ cup	100
Tempeh	½ cup	165
ACCEPTABLE		
Tofu, firm, raw	¼ block (about 3 oz)	118

• Foods that get less than 1 percent of their calories per serving from fat or saturated fat are designated by "<1."

• Unless otherwise specified, the foods are commercially prepared.

• While brand names are used in some cases, the nutrient information for many commercially prepared foods (such as frozen entrées) should be viewed as sample values. Expect variations among different brands and read labels carefully.

• Since beans, fruits and vegetables typically contain little or no saturated fat and cholesterol, we've devoted the most space to other food categories.

FAT (G)	SATURATED FAT (G)	% CALORIES FROM FAT	% CALORIES FROM SATURATED FAT	CHOLESTEROL (MG)
0.1	0.04	<1	<1	0
2	0.8	13.4	5.4	9
0.5	0.1	3.9	<1	0
0.3	0.1	2.9	1	0
1.4	0.1	8.8	<1	0
0.2	0.05	2.7	<1	0
0.4	0.1	3.2	<1	0
0.4	0.1	3.3	<1	0
1.4	0.5	9.3	3.3	0
0.2	0.04	8.2	1.6	0
7.7	1.1	46.5	6.6	0
2.4	0.3	48	6	0
0.4	0.1	3.1	<1	0
0.5	0	4.5	0	0
6.4	0.9	34.9	4.9	0
7.1	1	54.1	7.6	0

(continued)

Food	Portion	Calories
Beans, Bean Products and Other Legumes (cont.)		
High		
Chili, vegetarian, canned	1 cup	286
Chili with beans and meat, canned	1 cup	250
Breads and Bread Products		
Low		
Bagel, plain or onion	1 (about 2½ oz)	195
Blueberry muffin		
homemade with 2% milk	1 (about 2 oz)	163
low-fat, frozen	1 (about 2½ oz)	190
Breadstick, plain	1 (about ¼ oz)	25
Cornbread, homemade with 2% milk	1 piece (about 2¼ oz)	173
Corn muffin, homemade with 2% milk	1 (about 2 oz)	180
Cracked wheat bread	1 slice (about 1 oz)	65
English muffin, plain, toasted	1 (about 2 oz)	133
French, Vienna or sourdough bread	1 slice (about 1 oz)	69
Italian bread	1 slice (about 1 oz)	81
Pita bread, white	1 (about 2 oz)	165
Pumpernickel bread	1 slice (about 1 oz)	80
Raisin bread	1 slice (about 1 oz)	71
Roll or bun, homemade with whole milk	1 (about 1 oz)	112
Rye bread	1 slice (about 1 oz)	83
Wheat bread, reduced-calorie	1 slice (about 1 oz)	46
White bread, soft crumb	1 slice (about 1 oz)	67

Fat (g)	Saturated Fat (g)	% Calories from Fat	% Calories from Saturated Fat	Cholesterol (mg)
14	6	44.1	18.9	43
11	5	39.6	18	50
1.1	0.2	5.1	<1	0
6.2	1.2	34.2	6.6	21
5	1	23.7	4.7	5
0.6	0.1	21.6	3.6	0
4.6	1	23.9	5.2	26
7	1.3	35	6.5	24
1	0.2	13.8	2.8	0
1	0.2	6.8	1.4	0
0.8	0.2	10.4	2.6	0
1.1	0.3	12.2	3.3	0
0.7	0.1	3.8	<1	0
1	0.1	11.3	1.1	0
1.1	0.3	13.9	3.8	0
2.7	0.7	21.7	5.6	13
1.1	0.2	11.9	2.2	0
0.5	0.1	9.8	2	0
0.9	0.2	12.1	2.7	<1

(continued)

FOOD	PORTION	CALORIES

BREADS AND BREAD PRODUCTS (CONT.)

ACCEPTABLE

Biscuit, buttermilk, refrigerator	2 (about 2 oz total)	170
Bran muffin, homemade with wheat bran and 2% milk	1 (about 2 oz)	161
Cinnamon roll, refrigerator, baked, with frosting	1 (about 1 oz)	109
Zwieback rusks	5 pieces (about 1 oz)	149

HIGH

Biscuit, baking powder, homemade	1 (about 1 oz)	103
Croissant	1 (about 2 oz)	235
Popover, homemade	1 (about 1½ oz)	90
Spoon bread, homemade with vegetable shortening	1 cup	468

BREAKFAST FOODS

LOW

Danish, cinnamon nut (Arby's)	1 (3½ oz)	360
French toast, frozen, with low-calorie syrup	2 slices (about 4 oz total) with 4 Tbsp syrup	340
Hash browns, frozen, oven-heated	1 patty (about 2½ oz)	110
Pancakes with 2 pats butter and syrup (McDonald's)	3 (about 9 oz total)	560
Toaster pastry with fruit	1	204
Waffle, frozen, with low-calorie syrup	1 (about 1¼ oz) with 2 Tbsp syrup	136

ACCEPTABLE

Coffee cake, caramel nut	1 slice (about 2 oz)	240
Doughnut, plain, made without yeast	1 (about 2 oz)	198

HIGH

Biscuit with egg, cheese and sausage, frozen	1 (about 5½ oz)	490
Biscuit with egg and sausage (McDonald's)	1 (about 6½ oz)	520

Fat (g)	Saturated Fat (g)	% Calories from Fat	% Calories from Saturated Fat	Cholesterol (mg)
7	1.5	37.1	7.9	0
7	1.3	39.1	7.3	19
4	1	33	8.3	0
3.4	1.4	20.5	8.3	7
4.8	1.2	41.9	10.5	1
12	3.5	46	13.4	13
3.7	1.3	37	13	59
27.4	8.7	52.7	16.7	293
11	1	27.5	2.5	0
6	1.5	15.9	4	80
6	0	49.1	0	0
14	2.5	22.5	4	10
5.3	0.8	23.4	3.5	0
2.1	0.5	13.9	3.3	0
12	2.5	45	9.4	20
10.8	1.8	49.1	8.2	17
30	12	55.1	22	145
35	10	60.6	17.3	245

(continued)

FOOD	PORTION	CALORIES

BREAKFAST FOODS (CONT.)

HIGH (CONT.)

Croissant with egg, cheese and sausage (Burger King)	1 (about 6 oz)	530
Croissant with ham and cheese (Arby's)	1 (about 4¼ oz)	345
Danish, cheese (McDonald's)	1 (about 4 oz)	410
Doughnut, cream-filled, yeast or raised	1 (about 3 oz)	307
English muffin with egg, cheese and Canadian bacon (McDonald's)	1 (about 5 oz)	290
French toast sticks without butter and syrup (Burger King)	5 (about 5½ oz total)	500
Hash browns (McDonald's)	1 patty (about 2 oz)	130

COLD CEREALS

LOW

Cheerios with fat-free milk	1 cup with ½ cup milk	150
Granola without raisins, low-fat, with fat-free milk	½ cup with ½ cup milk	250
Kellogg's Frosted Flakes with fat-free milk	¾ cup with ½ cup milk	160
Raisin Bran with fat-free milk	1 cup with ½ cup milk	210
Shredded Wheat without milk	2 biscuits	160
Trix with fat-free milk	1 cup with ½ cup milk	160

ACCEPTABLE

| Cinnamon Toast Crunch with 2% milk | ¾ cup with ½ cup milk | 190 |

HIGH

| Cracklin' Oat Bran with fat-free milk | ¾ cup with ½ cup milk | 270 |
| 100% Natural with fruit and nuts, with 2% milk | ⅔ cup with ½ cup milk | 310 |

FAT (G)	SATURATED FAT (G)	% CALORIES FROM FAT	% CALORIES FROM SATURATED FAT	CHOLESTEROL (MG)
41	14	69.6	23.8	255
20.7	12.1	54	31.6	90
22	8	48.3	17.6	70
20.8	5.7	61	16.7	20
13	4.5	40.3	14	235
27	7	48.6	12.6	0
8	1.5	55.4	10.4	0
2	0.5	12	3	<5
3	0	10.8	0	0
0	0	0	0	0
1	0	4.3	0	0
0.5	0	2.8	0	0
1.5	0.5	8.4	2.8	<5
6	2	28.4	9.5	0
8	3	26.7	10	0
13.5	3.5	39.2	10.2	0

(continued)

FOOD	PORTION	CALORIES
BREAKFAST FOODS (CONT.)		
HOT CEREALS		
LOW		
Cream of Rice, cooked	³⁄₄ cup	95
Cream of Wheat, quick-cooking, cooked	³⁄₄ cup	97
Farina, enriched, cooked	³⁄₄ cup	88
Oatmeal, cooked	³⁄₄ cup	109
Ralston, cooked	³⁄₄ cup	101
Wheatena, cooked	³⁄₄ cup	102
CANDY AND SWEETS		
LOW		
Butterscotch	4 pieces (about 1 oz total)	112
Hard candy	3 pieces (about ¹⁄₂ oz total)	60
Marshmallow chicks	5 small (about 2 oz total)	160
Peanut brittle	1 piece (about 1¹⁄₃ oz)	180
ACCEPTABLE		
Fudge, vanilla, homemade	1 piece (about 1 oz)	105
HIGH		
Almonds, chocolate-coated	7 (about 1 oz total)	159
Caramels	3 (about 1 oz total)	108
Chocolate bar, semisweet	1 (about 1¹⁄₂ oz)	230
Coconut bar, chocolate-coated	1 (about 2 oz)	195
Fudge, chocolate with nuts, homemade	1 piece (about 1 oz)	121
Mints, chocolate-coated	2 (about ¹⁄₃ oz total)	29
Peanuts, chocolate-coated	10 (about 1¹⁄₂ oz total)	208
Raisins, chocolate-coated	10 (about ¹⁄₃ oz total)	39
Vanilla creams, chocolate-coated	1 oz	122

Fat (G)	Saturated Fat (G)	% Calories from Fat	% Calories from Saturated Fat	Cholesterol (MG)
0.2	0	1.9	0	0
0.4	0	3.7	0	0
0.2	0.02	2	<1	0
1.8	0.3	14.9	2.5	0
0.6	0	5.3	0	0
0.9	0	7.9	0	0
1	0.3	8	2.4	3
0	0	0	0	0
0	0	0	0	0
5	1	25	5	0
1.5	1	12.9	8.6	5
12.2	2.1	69.1	11.9	0
2.3	1.9	19.2	15.8	2
13	9	50.9	35.2	10
11.7	6.2	54	28.6	0
4.6	1.6	34.2	11.9	4
1.1	0.7	34.1	21.7	0
13.4	5.8	58	25.1	4
1.5	0.9	34.6	20.8	1
4.8	1.4	35.4	10.3	1

(continued)

FOOD	PORTION	CALORIES
CHEESE AND CHEESE PRODUCTS		
LOW		
American, fat-free	1 slice (about ¾ oz)	30
Cheddar, fat-free	1 oz	45
Cream cheese, fat-free	2 Tbsp	30
Swiss, fat-free	1 slice (about ¾ oz)	30
Yogurt cheese, low-fat	1 oz	30
ACCEPTABLE		
Cottage cheese, 1%	½ cup	82
HIGH		
American	1 oz	106
Blue cheese	1 oz	99
Brie	1 oz	93
Camembert	1 oz	84
Caraway	1 oz	105
Cheddar		
reduced-fat	1 oz	80
regular	1 oz	110
Colby	1 oz	110
Cottage cheese		
creamed, small or large curd	½ cup	109
2%	½ cup	101
Cream cheese		
reduced-fat	2 Tbsp	70
regular	1 oz	100
Feta	1 oz	74
Fondue	¼ cup	151
Gouda	1 oz	100
Gruyère	1 oz	116
Limburger	1 oz	92
Monterey Jack	1 oz	105
Mozzarella		
reduced-fat	1 oz	71
regular	1 oz	79

Fat (g)	Saturated Fat (g)	% Calories from Fat	% Calories from Saturated Fat	Cholesterol (mg)
0	0	0	0	0
0	0	0	0	25
0	0	0	0	5
0	0	0	0	0
0.6	Trace	18	Trace	0
1.2	0.7	13.2	7.7	5
8.9	5.6	75.6	47.5	27
8.1	5.2	73.6	47.3	21
7.6	4.9	73.5	47.4	28
6.8	4.3	72.9	46.1	20
8.2	5.2	70.3	44.6	26
5	3	56.3	33.8	20
9	6	73.6	49	30
9	5.7	73.6	46.6	27
4.7	3	38.8	24.8	16
2.2	1.4	19.6	12.5	10
5	3.5	64.3	45	15
10	6	90	54	30
6	4.2	72.9	51.1	25
10.4	5.1	62	30.4	128
7.7	4.9	69.3	44.1	32
9.1	5.3	70.6	41.1	31
7.6	4.7	74.3	46	25
8.5	5.3	72.9	45.4	25
4.5	2.8	57	35.5	16
6.1	3.7	69.5	42.2	22

(continued)

FOOD	PORTION	CALORIES

CHEESE AND CHEESE PRODUCTS (CONT.)

HIGH (CONT.)

Muenster		
reduced-fat	1 oz	80
regular	1 oz	103
Neufchâtel	1 oz	73
Parmesan, grated	1 Tbsp	23
Provolone	1 oz	98
Ricotta		
reduced-fat	½ cup	171
regular	½ cup	216
Romano, grated	1 Tbsp	19
Soufflé, homemade	1 cup	207
Swiss	1 oz	105
Welsh rarebit, frozen	¼ cup (about 2 oz)	120

DESSERTS

CAKES

LOW

Angel food	1 slice (¹/₁₂ of cake)	73
Fruitcake	1 slice (about 2 oz)	139
Sponge	1 slice (¹/₁₂ of cake)	110

ACCEPTABLE

Boston cream	1 slice (¹/₆ of cake)	232
Devil's food, made from mix with eggs and oil, with 2 Tbsp chocolate icing	1 slice (¹/₁₂ of cake)	440
Pound, made with margarine	1 slice (¹/₁₆ of loaf cake)	206
White, made from mix with egg whites and oil, with 2 Tbsp reduced-calorie chocolate icing	1 slice (¹/₁₂ of cake)	370

Fat (g)	Saturated Fat (g)	% Calories from Fat	% Calories from Saturated Fat	Cholesterol (mg)
5	**3**	56.3	**33.8**	20
8.4	**5.4**	73.4	**47.2**	27
6.6	**4.1**	81.4	**50.5**	21
1.5	**1**	58.7	**39.1**	4
7.5	**4.8**	68.9	**44.1**	19
9.8	**6.1**	51.6	**32.1**	38
16.1	**10.3**	67.1	**42.9**	63
1.4	**0.9**	66.3	**42.6**	5
16.2	**8.2**	70.4	**35.7**	176
7.7	**5**	66	**42.9**	26
9	**4**	67.5	**30**	20
0.2	**0.03**	2.5	**<1**	0
3.9	**0.5**	25.3	**3.2**	2
1	**0.3**	8.2	**2.5**	39
7.8	**2.3**	30.3	**8.9**	35
21	**4.5**	43	**9.2**	45
9	**1.9**	39.3	**8.3**	41
11	**3**	26.8	**7.3**	0

(continued)

FOOD	PORTION	CALORIES

DESSERTS (CONT.)

CAKES (CONT.)

HIGH

Carrot cake, homemade with cream cheese icing	1 slice ($^1/_{12}$ of cake)	484
Cheesecake, frozen	$^1/_4$ cake (about 4$^1/_4$ oz)	350
Pound, made with butter	1 slice ($^1/_{12}$ of cake)	110
Yellow with pudding, made from mix with eggs and margarine, with 2 Tbsp chocolate icing	1 slice ($^1/_{12}$ of cake)	410

COOKIES

LOW

Brownie with nuts, made from mix	1 (about $^3/_4$ oz)	81
Fig bars, fat-free	2 (about 1 oz total)	100
Gingersnaps	5 (about 1$^1/_4$ oz total)	147
Ladyfingers	4 (about 1$^1/_2$ oz total)	158
Molasses	2 (about 2 oz total)	274
Oatmeal with raisins		
homemade	1 (about $^1/_2$ oz)	65
reduced-fat	2 (about 1 oz total)	110

ACCEPTABLE

Fig bars	2 (about 1 oz total)	110
Peanut butter, homemade	1 (about $^3/_4$ oz)	95
Sugar, homemade with margarine	1 (about $^1/_2$ oz)	66

HIGH

Chocolate chip, homemade with margarine	1 (about $^1/_2$ oz)	78
Macaroon, homemade	1 (about 1 oz)	97
Sandwich, vanilla with cream filling	4 (about 2 oz total)	297
Sugar wafer with cream filling	1 small	18
Vanilla wafers	8 (about 1 oz total)	150

FAT (G)	SATURATED FAT (G)	% CALORIES FROM FAT	% CALORIES FROM SATURATED FAT	CHOLESTEROL (MG)
29.3	5.4	54.5	10	60
18	9	46.3	23.1	50
5.6	3.2	45.8	26.2	63
17	7.5	37.3	16.5	75
3.7	0.6	41.1	6.6	13
0	0	0	0	0
3.1	0.8	19	4.9	14
3.4	1.1	19.4	6.7	157
6.9	1.7	22.7	5.6	25
2.4	0.5	33.2	6.9	5
2.5	0	20.5	0	0
2.5	1	20.5	8.2	0
4.8	0.9	45.5	8.5	6
3.3	0.7	45	9.5	4
4.5	1.3	51.9	15	5
3.1	2.7	28.8	25.1	0
13.5	3.7	41	11.2	23
0.9	0.2	45	10	0
7	2	42	12	0

(continued)

FOOD	PORTION	CALORIES

DESSERTS (CONT.)

PIES

LOW

| Apple, low-fat, frozen | 1 slice (⅕ of pie) | 220 |
| Pecan, fresh | 1 slice (⅛ of pie) | 431 |

ACCEPTABLE

| Rhubarb, fresh | 1 slice (⅛ of pie) | 299 |

HIGH

Apple, fresh	1 slice (⅛ of pie)	302
Banana custard, fresh	1 slice (⅛ of pie)	252
Blueberry, fresh	1 slice (⅛ of pie)	286
Cherry, fresh	1 slice (⅛ of pie)	308
Chocolate meringue, fresh	1 slice (⅛ of pie)	287
Custard, fresh	1 slice (⅛ of pie)	249
Lemon meringue, fresh	1 slice (⅛ of pie)	268
Mince, fresh	1 slice (⅛ of pie)	320
Pumpkin, fresh	1 slice (⅛ of pie)	241

PUDDING

ACCEPTABLE

| Vanilla, made from mix with 2% milk | ½ cup | 148 |

HIGH

Chocolate, made from mix with whole milk	½ cup	163
Custard, homemade, baked	½ cup	148
Rice with raisins, homemade	½ cup	194
Tapioca, made from mix with whole milk	½ cup	161

OTHER

LOW

| Fruit cocktail, canned in light syrup | ½ cup | 72 |
| Gelatin, made from powder, with fruit | ½ cup | 80 |

Fat (g)	Saturated Fat (g)	% Calories from Fat	% Calories from Saturated Fat	Cholesterol (mg)
5	1	20.5	4.1	0
23.6	3.3	49.3	6.9	65
12.6	3.1	37.9	9.3	0
13.1	3.4	39	10.1	0
10.6	3.4	37.9	12.1	66
12.7	3.2	40	10.1	0
13.3	3.5	38.9	10.2	0
13.7	5.1	43	16	64
12.7	4.3	45.9	15.5	120
10.7	3.2	35.9	10.7	98
13.6	3.6	38.3	10.1	1
12.8	4.5	47.8	16.8	70
2.4	1.4	14.6	8.5	9
4.6	2.7	25.4	14.9	16
6.6	3.3	40.1	20.1	123
4.1	2.2	19	10.2	15
4.1	2.5	22.9	14	17
0.1	0.01	1.3	<1	0
0.1	0	1.1	0	0

(continued)

FOOD	PORTION	CALORIES

DESSERTS (CONT.)

OTHER (CONT.)

HIGH

Coconut cream, canned	½ cup	142
Eclair	1 (about 3½ oz)	239

DIPS AND SNACKS

DIPS

LOW

Hummus	⅓ cup	140
Onion, low-fat	2 Tbsp	30
Salsa	2 Tbsp	10

HIGH

Bacon and horseradish	2 Tbsp	60
Cheese		
low-fat	2 Tbsp	80
regular	2 Tbsp	90
Clam	2 Tbsp	50
Onion	2 Tbsp	60
Ranch	2 Tbsp	140

SNACKS

LOW

Caramel corn	½ cup	140
Cereal mix	¾ cup	130
Cracker Jacks	1 box	150
Crackers		
graham	1 (½ oz)	55
saltines	5 (½ oz total)	61
Crispbread, rye	1 slice	35
Fruit rolls	2	110

Fat (g)	Saturated Fat (g)	% Calories from Fat	% Calories from Saturated Fat	Cholesterol (mg)
13.1	**11.6**	83	**73.5**	0
13.6	**4.4**	51.2	**16.6**	136
6.9	**1**	44.4	**6.4**	0
0	**0**	0	**0**	<5
0	**0**	0	**0**	0
5	**3**	75	**45**	20
3	**2**	33.6	**22.5**	15
7	**5**	70	**50**	20
4.5	**3**	81	**54**	20
5	**3**	75	**45**	20
14	**2.5**	90	**16.1**	10
4	**1**	25.7	**6.4**	<5
5	**1**	34.6	**6.9**	0
3	**0.5**	18	**3**	0
1.3	**0.3**	21.3	**4.9**	0
1.7	**0.4**	25.1	**5.9**	0
0	**0**	0	**0**	0
1	**Trace**	8.2	**Trace**	0

(continued)

FOOD	PORTION	CALORIES

DIPS AND SNACKS (CONT.)

SNACKS (CONT.)

LOW (CONT.)

Granola bar, chocolate chip, low-fat	1 (about 1 oz)	110
Melba toast	3 pieces (about ½ oz total)	55
Popcorn		
air-popped, plain	1 cup	31
microwave, butter-flavored, light	1 bag (about 13 cups)	110
Potato chips, fat-free	30 (about 1 oz total)	110
Pretzels		
baked	16 (about 1 oz total)	120
cheese-flavored	1 oz	160
Dutch-type	2 large (about 1 oz total)	125
Rice cakes, flavored	1 (about ½ oz)	50
Toffee corn (popcorn and peanuts)	⅔ cup (about 1 oz)	140
Tortilla chips, plain	13 (about 1 oz total)	140

ACCEPTABLE

Corn chips	30 small (about 1 oz total)	155
Popcorn, microwave		
butter-flavored	1 bag (about 13 cups)	150
plain	1 bag (about 13 cups)	140

HIGH

Cheez Doodles	17 (about 1 oz total)	150
Crackers		
butter-flavored	4 (about ½ oz total)	64
cheese	4 round (½ oz total)	67
cheese and peanut butter	2 (½ oz total)	69
wheat	7 (½ oz total)	61
Granola bar, chocolate chip	1 (about 1 oz)	120

Fat (g)	Saturated Fat (g)	% Calories from Fat	% Calories from Saturated Fat	Cholesterol (mg)
2	0.5	16.4	4.1	0
0.5	0.1	8.2	1.6	0
0.3	0.1	8.7	2.9	0
4	0.5	32.7	4.1	0
0	0	0	0	0
2.5	0	18.8	0	0
7	1	39.4	5.6	0
1.4	0.3	10.1	2.2	0
0	0	0	0	0
4	1	25.7	6.4	<5
6	1	38.6	6.4	0
9.1	1.5	52.8	8.7	0
10	1.5	60	9	0
10	1.5	64.3	9.6	0
8	2.5	48	15	0
2.5	0.8	35.2	11.3	0
3	1.2	40.2	16.1	4
3.4	0.9	44.3	11.7	2
1.8	0.9	26.6	13.3	0
3.5	1.5	26.3	11.3	0

(continued)

FOOD	PORTION	CALORIES
DIPS AND SNACKS (CONT.)		
SNACKS (CONT.)		
HIGH (CONT.)		
Popcorn, buttered	1 cup	41
Potato chips	10 (about ¾ oz total)	105
Potato sticks	1 oz	148
Sesame sticks	30 pieces (about 1 oz total)	170
Wheat Nuts (wheat germ nuggets)	1 oz	200
DRESSINGS		
LOW		
Blue cheese, fat-free	2 Tbsp	35
Caesar, low-fat	2 Tbsp	70
French, fat-free	2 Tbsp	50
Garlic, creamy, fat-free	2 Tbsp	40
Honey dijon, fat-free	2 Tbsp	50
Italian		
low-fat	2 Tbsp	15
fat-free	2 Tbsp	15
Oil and vinegar, imitation, fat-free	2 Tbsp	15
Ranch		
low-fat	2 Tbsp	80
fat-free	2 Tbsp	45
Thousand Island		
low-fat	2 Tbsp	45
fat-free	2 Tbsp	35
ACCEPTABLE		
French, low-fat	2 Tbsp	50
Ranch	2 Tbsp	140
Russian	2 Tbsp	110

Fat (g)	Saturated Fat (g)	% Calories from Fat	% Calories from Saturated Fat	Cholesterol (mg)
2	0.9	43.9	19.8	4
7.1	1.8	60.9	15.4	0
9.8	2.5	59.6	15.2	0
12	2	63.5	10.6	0
19	3	85.5	13.5	0
0	0	0	0	0
6	0.5	77.1	6.4	5
0	0	0	0	0
0	0	0	0	0
0	0	0	0	0
0.5	0	30	0	0
0	0	0	0	0
0	0	0	0	0
7	0.5	78.8	5.6	0
0	0	0	0	0
1	0	20	0	<5
0	0	0	0	0
3	0.5	54	9	0
14	1.5	90	9.6	10
6	1	49.1	8.2	0

(continued)

FOOD	PORTION	CALORIES
DRESSINGS (CONT.)		
HIGH		
Blue cheese		
low-fat	2 Tbsp	80
regular	2 Tbsp	170
Caesar	2 Tbsp	170
French	2 Tbsp	120
Garlic, creamy	2 Tbsp	140
Honey dijon	2 Tbsp	130
Italian	2 Tbsp	100
Italian, creamy		
low-fat	2 Tbsp	50
regular	2 Tbsp	110
Oil and vinegar		
low-fat	2 Tbsp	60
regular	2 Tbsp	110
Sweet-and-sour	2 Tbsp	150
Thousand Island	2 Tbsp	110
EGGS AND EGG SUBSTITUTE		
LOW		
Egg white	1 large	16
ACCEPTABLE		
Egg substitute, liquid	¼ cup	53
HIGH		
Egg		
fried with margarine	1 large	92
hard-boiled	1 large	78
scrambled with butter and whole milk	1 large	95
Egg substitute, frozen	¼ cup	96
Egg yolk	1 large	59

Fat (g)	Saturated Fat (g)	% Calories from Fat	% Calories from Saturated Fat	Cholesterol (mg)
8	2	90	22.5	0
17	3	90	15.9	10
18	2.5	95.3	13.2	0
12	2	90	15	0
13	2	83.6	12.9	0
10	1.5	69.2	10.4	0
10	1.5	90	13.5	0
5	1	90	18	0
11	4	90	32.7	0
5	1	75	15	0
11	2	90	16.4	0
13	2	78	12	0
10	1.5	81.8	12.3	10
Trace	0	Trace	0	0
2.1	0.4	35.7	7	1
6.9	1.9	67.5	18.6	211
5.3	1.6	61.2	18.5	212
7.1	2.8	67.3	26.5	248
6.7	1.2	62.8	11.3	1
5.1	1.6	77.8	24.4	213

(continued)

FOOD	PORTION	CALORIES

EGGS AND EGG SUBSTITUTE (CONT.)

HIGH (CONT.)

Quiche

Lorraine	1 slice (about 6¼ oz)	600
spinach, frozen	1 (about 6 oz)	480

FAST FOODS

LOW

Baked potato with cheese and bacon (Wendy's)	1 (about 10 oz)	530
BBQ Beef sandwich on bun (Dairy Queen/Brazier)	1 (about 4 oz)	225
Fish, breaded, baked, without bun (Long John Silver's)	3 pieces (about 5 oz total)	150
Onion rings, breaded (Burger King)	1 order (about 5 oz)	310

ACCEPTABLE

Baked potato with sour cream and chives (Wendy's)	1 (about 10 oz)	380
Burrito, bean (Taco Bell)	1	391
Chicken, breaded, with mayonnaise, lettuce and tomato on bun (Wendy's)	1 (about 9 oz)	450
Chicken breast and wing quarter, roasted, without skin (KFC)	(about 4 oz total)	199
Fish, breaded, with tartar sauce on bun (McDonald's)	1 (about 6 oz)	360
French fries (McDonald's)	1 large (about 6 oz)	450
Garden salad with 2 Tbsp reduced-fat, reduced-calorie Italian dressing (Wendy's)	1 (about 10 oz)	150
Pie, apple (Burger King)	1 (about 4 oz)	310
Shake, chocolate (McDonald's)	1 small (about 16 oz)	350

HIGH

Baked potato with chili and cheese (Wendy's)	1 (about 10 oz)	610

Fat (G)	Saturated Fat (G)	% Calories from Fat	% Calories from Saturated Fat	Cholesterol (MG)
48	**23.2**	72	**34.8**	285
32	**16**	60	**30**	205
18	**4**	30.6	**6.8**	20
4	**1**	16	**4**	20
1	**0.6**	6	**3.6**	110
14	**2**	40.6	**5.8**	0
6	**4**	14.2	**9.5**	15
12	**4**	27.6	**9.2**	5
20	**4**	40	**8**	60
5.9	**1.7**	26.7	**7.7**	97
16	**3.5**	40	**8.8**	35
22	**4**	44	**8**	0
9	**1.5**	54	**9**	0
15	**3**	43.5	**8.7**	0
6	**3.5**	15.4	**9**	25
24	**9**	35.4	**13.3**	45

(continued)

FOOD	PORTION	CALORIES

FAST FOODS (CONT.)

HIGH (CONT.)

Baked potato with broccoli and cheese (Arby's)	1 (about 10 oz)	417
Burrito, chicken (Taco Bell)	1	345
Cheeseburger with condiments on bun (Burger King)	1 (about 5 oz)	320
Cheese steak with onions and peppers on bun (Arby's)	1 (about 7 oz)	467
Chef's salad with turkey, ham, cheese and Thousand Island dressing (Arby's)	1 (about 14 oz)	503
Chicken breast, fried (KFC)	1 (about 5 oz)	360
Chicken nuggets without sauce (KFC)	6 (about 3 oz total)	284
Double cheeseburger with condiments on bun (Burger King)	1 (about 8 oz)	600
Hamburger with condiments on bun (McDonald's)	1 (about 4 oz)	270
Hot dog, plain, on bun (Dairy Queen/ Brazier)	1 (about 3 oz)	280
Nachos Supreme (Taco Bell)	1 order	364
Roast beef on bun (Arby's)	1 (about 6 oz)	383
Shake, vanilla (McDonald's)	1 small (about 16 oz)	310
Submarine		
Italian (cold cuts) (Arby's)	1 (about 10 oz)	671
Tuna (Arby's)	1 (about 10 oz)	663
Taco, beef (Taco Bell)	1	180
Taco salad with small chili and 1 packet sour cream (Wendy's)	1 (about 30 oz)	830
Tostada (Taco Bell)	1	242

Fat (G)	Saturated Fat (G)	% Calories from Fat	% Calories from Saturated Fat	Cholesterol (MG)
17.9	6.9	38.6	14.9	22
13	5	33.9	13	57
13	6	36.6	16.9	40
25.3	9.7	48.8	18.7	53
38.7	8.2	69.2	14.7	150
20	5	50	12.5	115
18	4	57	12.7	68
36	17	54	25.5	135
9	3	30	10	30
16	6	51.4	19.3	25
18	5	44.5	12.4	17
18.2	7	42.8	16.4	43
5	3.5	14.5	10.2	25
38.8	12.8	52	17.2	69
37	8.2	50.2	11.1	43
11	5	55	25	32
42	17.5	45.5	19	125
11	4	40.9	14.9	14

(continued)

FOOD	PORTION	CALORIES

FATS, OILS AND SPREADS

FATS

HIGH
Chicken	1 Tbsp	115
Lard	1 Tbsp	115
Shortening	1 Tbsp	113

OILS

ACCEPTABLE
Almond	1 Tbsp	120
Canola	1 Tbsp	124
Grapeseed	1 Tbsp	120
Safflower	1 Tbsp	120
Walnut	1 Tbsp	120

HIGH
Avocado	1 Tbsp	124
Coconut	1 Tbsp	120
Corn	1 Tbsp	120
Cottonseed	1 Tbsp	120
Olive	1 Tbsp	119
Palm	1 Tbsp	120
Peanut	1 Tbsp	119
Sesame	1 Tbsp	120
Soybean	1 Tbsp	120
Sunflower	1 Tbsp	120

SPREADS

LOW
Apple butter	1 Tbsp	33
Mayonnaise, low-fat	1 Tbsp	25

Fat (G)	Saturated Fat (G)	% Calories from Fat	% Calories from Saturated Fat	Cholesterol (MG)
12.8	3.8	100	29.7	11
12.8	5	100	39.1	4
12.8	3.2	100	25.5	0
13.6	1.1	100	8.3	0
14	1	100	7.3	0
13.6	1.3	100	9.8	0
13.6	1.2	100	9	0
13.6	1.2	100	9	0
14	1.6	100	11.6	0
13.6	11.8	100	88.5	0
13.6	1.7	100	12.8	0
13.6	3.5	100	26.3	0
13.5	1.8	100	13.6	0
13.6	6.7	100	50.3	0
13.5	2.3	100	17.4	0
13.6	1.9	100	14.3	0
13.6	2	100	15	0
13.6	1.4	100	10.5	0
0.1	0	2.7	0	0
1	0	36	0	0

(continued)

FOOD	PORTION	CALORIES

FATS, OILS AND SPREADS (CONT.)

SPREADS (CONT.)

ACCEPTABLE

Almond butter, unsalted	1 Tbsp	101
Peanut butter without added oils	2 Tbsp	200

HIGH

Butter, salted, unsalted stick or whipped	1 Tbsp	102
Butter blend, made with butter and vegetable oil	1 Tbsp	50
Margarine		
squeeze	1 Tbsp	80
stick		
reduced-fat	1 Tbsp	60
regular	1 Tbsp	100
tub		
reduced-fat	1 Tbsp	45
regular	1 Tbsp	100
Mayonnaise		
reduced-fat	1 Tbsp	50
regular	1 Tbsp	100
Peanut butter with added oils, smooth	2 Tbsp	188

FISH AND SHELLFISH

FISH

LOW

Bass, striped, uncooked	3 oz	82
Bluefish, uncooked	3 oz	105
Cod, Atlantic, broiled, baked or microwaved	3 oz	89
Flounder, broiled, baked or microwaved	3 oz	99
Grouper, broiled, baked or microwaved	3 oz	100
Haddock, broiled, baked or microwaved	3 oz	95
Halibut, broiled, baked or microwaved	3 oz	119

Fat (g)	Saturated Fat (g)	% Calories from Fat	% Calories from Saturated Fat	Cholesterol (mg)
9.5	0.9	84.7	8	0
16	2	72	9	0
11.5	7.2	100	63.5	31
6	3	100	54	10
9	1.5	100	16.9	0
6	1	90	15	0
11	2	99	18	0
4.5	1	90	20	0
11	2	99	18	0
5	1	90	18	5
11	1.5	99	13.5	5
16	3.1	76.6	14.8	0
2	0.4	22	4.4	68
3.6	0.8	30.9	6.9	50
0.7	0.1	7.1	1	47
1.3	0.3	11.8	2.7	58
1.1	0.3	9.9	2.7	40
0.8	0.1	7.6	<1	63
2.5	0.4	18.9	3	35

(continued)

FOOD	PORTION	CALORIES

FISH AND SHELLFISH (CONT.)

FISH (CONT.)

LOW (CONT.)

Mahimahi, uncooked	3 oz	72
Monkfish, uncooked	3 oz	65
Ocean perch, Atlantic, broiled, baked or microwaved	3 oz	103
Orange roughy, broiled, baked or microwaved	3 oz	75
Pollack, broiled, baked or microwaved	3 oz	96
Shark, mixed species, uncooked	3 oz	111
Smelt, rainbow, broiled, baked or microwaved	3 oz	105
Snapper, mixed species, broiled, baked or microwaved	3 oz	109
Sole, broiled, baked or microwaved	3 oz	99
Surimi, uncooked	3 oz	84
Trout, rainbow, broiled, baked or microwaved	3 oz	128
Tuna, light meat, canned in water	3 oz	99
Turbot, European, uncooked	3 oz	81
Whitefish, mixed species, smoked	3 oz	92

ACCEPTABLE

Anchovies, canned in olive oil	5 (about ¾ oz total)	42
Carp, broiled, baked or microwaved	3 oz	138
Salmon		
pink, canned, with bones and liquid	3 oz	118
sockeye, fresh, broiled, baked or microwaved	3 oz	184
Sardines, Atlantic, canned in oil, drained, with bones	2 (about 1 oz total)	50
Swordfish, broiled, baked or microwaved	3 oz	132
Tuna, fresh, broiled, baked or microwaved	3 oz	156
Tuna salad, prepared with mayonnaise	3 oz	159

Fat (G)	Saturated Fat (G)	% Calories from Fat	% Calories from Saturated Fat	Cholesterol (MG)
0.6	0.2	7.5	2.5	62
1.3	0.3	18	4.2	21
1.8	0.3	15.7	2.6	46
0.8	0.02	9.6	<1	22
1	0.2	9.4	1.9	82
3.8	0.8	30.8	6.5	43
2.6	0.5	22.3	4.3	77
1.5	0.3	12.4	2.5	40
1.3	0.3	11.8	2.7	58
0.7	0.2	7.5	2.1	26
3.7	0.7	26	4.9	62
0.7	0.2	6.4	1.8	26
2.5	0.6	27.8	6.7	41
0.8	0.2	7.8	2	28
1.9	0.4	40.7	8.6	17
6.1	1.2	39.8	7.8	71
5.1	1.3	38.9	9.9	47
9.3	1.6	45.5	7.8	74
2.8	0.4	50.4	7.2	34
4.4	1.2	30	8.2	43
5.3	1.4	30.6	8.1	42
7.9	1.3	44.7	7.4	11

(continued)

FOOD	PORTION	CALORIES

FISH AND SHELLFISH (CONT.)

FISH (CONT.)

HIGH

Catfish, channel, breaded and fried	3 oz	195
Caviar, black or red	1 Tbsp	40
Eel, broiled, baked or microwaved	3 oz	201
Herring, kippered	1 fillet (about 1½ oz)	87
Mackerel, Atlantic, broiled, baked or microwaved	3 oz	223
Pompano, Florida, broiled, baked or microwaved	3 oz	179

SHELLFISH

LOW

Clams, steamed	20 small (about 3 oz)	133
Crab, Alaskan king, steamed	3 oz	82
Crayfish (crawfish), steamed	3 oz	97
Lobster, boiled, poached or steamed	3 oz	83
Mussels, blue, boiled, poached or steamed	3 oz	146
Scallops, uncooked	3 oz	75
Shrimp, mixed species, steamed	3 oz	84

ACCEPTABLE

Lobster salad, prepared with mayonnaise	½ cup	286
Oysters, eastern, steamed	6 medium (about 1½ oz total)	57
Shrimp, mixed species, breaded and fried	3 oz	206

HIGH

Clams, mixed species, breaded and fried	20 small (about 6¾ oz total)	380
Crab, soft-shell, fried	1 (about 4½ oz)	334
Oysters, Eastern, breaded and fried	6 medium (about 3 oz total)	173
Scallops, mixed species, breaded and fried	2 large (about 1 oz total)	67

Fat (G)	Saturated Fat (G)	% Calories from Fat	% Calories from Saturated Fat	Cholesterol (MG)
11.3	2.8	52.2	12.9	69
2.9	0.7	65.3	15.6	94
12.7	2.6	56.9	11.6	137
5	1.1	51.7	11.4	33
15.1	3.6	60.9	14.5	64
10.3	3.8	51.8	19.1	54
1.8	0.2	12.2	1.4	60
1.3	0.1	14.3	1.1	45
1.2	0.2	11.1	1.9	151
0.5	0.1	5.4	1.1	61
3.8	0.7	23.4	4.3	48
0.7	0.1	8.4	1.2	28
0.9	0.3	9.8	3.2	166
16.6	2.6	52.2	8.2	120
2.1	0.6	33.2	9.5	44
10.4	1.8	45.4	7.9	151
21	5	49.7	11.8	115
17.9	4.4	48.2	11.9	45
11.1	2.8	57.7	14.6	71
3.4	0.8	45.7	10.7	19

(continued)

FOOD	PORTION	CALORIES

FRUITS AND FRUIT JUICES

LOW

Apple, raw, with skin	1 (about 5 oz)	81
Apple juice, unsweetened, canned or bottled	1 cup	117
Cherries, sweet, without pits	1 cup	104
Figs, dried	3 (about 2 oz total)	145
Grapefruit, pink	½ (about 4 oz)	37
Grapes, green or red	1 cup	114
Orange juice, frozen, from concentrate	1 cup	112
Peach, raw	1 (about 3 oz)	37
Pears, canned in light syrup	½ cup	72
Raisins, seedless	½ cup	218
Strawberries	1 cup	45

HIGH

Avocado	½ (about 3 oz)	162

GRAINS

LOW

Barley, pearled, cooked	½ cup	97
Bran		
oat, raw	2 Tbsp	29
wheat, raw	2 Tbsp	15
Buckwheat groats, cooked	½ cup	91
Bulgur wheat, cooked	½ cup	76
Corn grits, white or yellow, cooked	½ cup	73
Cornmeal, whole grain, white or yellow, raw	¼ cup	109
Couscous, cooked	½ cup	101
Hominy, white or yellow, canned, raw	½ cup	58
Millet, cooked	½ cup	143
Quinoa, raw	¼ cup	159
Rye, raw	¼ cup	141
Wheat germ, toasted	¼ cup	108

Fat (G)	Saturated Fat (G)	% Calories from Fat	% Calories from Saturated Fat	Cholesterol (MG)
0.5	0.1	5.5	1.1	0
0.3	0.1	2.3	<1	0
1.4	0.3	12.1	2.6	0
0.7	0.1	4.3	<1	0
0.1	0.02	2.4	<1	0
0.9	0.3	7.1	2.4	0
0.2	0.02	1.6	<1	0
0.1	0.01	2.4	<1	0
0.04	0	<1	0	0
0.3	0.1	1.2	<1	0
0.6	0.03	12	<1	0
15.4	2.5	85.6	13.9	0
0.4	0.1	3.7	<1	0
0.8	0.2	24.8	6.2	0
0.3	0.04	18	2.4	0
0.6	0.1	6	<1	0
0.2	0.04	2.4	<1	0
0.2	0.04	2.5	<1	0
1.1	0.2	9.1	1.7	0
0.1	0.03	<1	<1	0
0.7	0.1	10.9	1.6	0
1.2	0.2	7.5	1.3	0
2.5	0.3	14.2	1.7	0
1.1	0.1	7	<1	0
3	0.5	25	4.2	0

(continued)

Food	Portion	Calories
Grains (cont.)		
High		
Bran, rice, raw	2 Tbsp	33
Rice		
Low		
Brown, cooked	½ cup	109
Chicken-flavored, made from mix with 2 Tbsp margarine (Rice-A-Roni)	1 cup	320
Fried, made from mix with 2 Tbsp margarine (Rice-A-Roni)	1 cup	320
Spanish, homemade	½ cup	107
White		
enriched, cooked	½ cup	133
instant, cooked	½ cup	80
Wild, cooked	½ cup	83
Gravies and Sauces		
Gravies		
Low		
Mushroom, canned	¼ cup	30
Onion, dry mix, prepared	¼ cup	20
Acceptable		
Au jus, canned	¼ cup	10
Brown, dry mix, prepared	¼ cup	19
High		
Beef, canned	¼ cup	31
Chicken, canned	¼ cup	47
Turkey, canned	¼ cup	30

Fat (g)	Saturated Fat (g)	% Calories from Fat	% Calories from Saturated Fat	Cholesterol (mg)
2.2	**0.4**	60	**10.9**	0
0.9	**0.2**	7.4	**1.7**	0
9.5	**1**	26.7	**2.8**	0
11	**2**	30.9	**5.6**	0
2.1	**0**	17.7	**0**	0
0.3	**0.1**	2	**<1**	0
0.1	**0.04**	1.1	**<1**	0
0.3	**0.04**	3.3	**<1**	0
1.6	**0.2**	48	**6**	0
0.2	**0.1**	9	**4.5**	0
0.1	**0.1**	9	**9**	0
0.4	**0.2**	18.9	**9.5**	1
1.4	**0.7**	40.6	**20.3**	2
3.4	**0.8**	65.1	**15.3**	1
1.3	**0.4**	39	**12**	1

(continued)

FOOD	PORTION	CALORIES

GRAVIES AND SAUCES (CONT.)

SAUCES

LOW

Barbecue, bottled	¼ cup	47
Marinara, canned	½ cup	85
Soy, tamari, bottled	1 Tbsp	11
Spaghetti, canned	½ cup	136
Sweet-and-sour, dry mix, made with water and vinegar	¼ cup	74
Teriyaki, bottled	¼ cup	60
Tomato, canned	1 cup	74
Worcestershire, bottled	1 tsp	0

HIGH

Alfredo, canned	½ cup	310
Bernaise, dry mix, made with milk and butter	¼ cup	175
Curry, dry mix, made with milk	¼ cup	67
Hollandaise, dry mix, made with milk and butter	¼ cup	176
Tartar	1 Tbsp	74
White		
dry mix, made with milk	¼ cup	60
medium, homemade	¼ cup	101

ICE CREAM AND FROZEN TREATS

LOW

Frozen yogurt, vanilla, fat-free	½ cup	110
Fruit ice	1 cup	247
Fruit juice bar	1 (about 1¾ oz)	42

ACCEPTABLE

Frozen yogurt, vanilla	½ cup	110
Ice cream, vanilla, low-fat	½ cup	100
Sherbet, orange	½ cup	135
Tofutti, all flavors	½ cup	217

Fat (G)	Saturated Fat (G)	% Calories from Fat	% Calories from Saturated Fat	Cholesterol (MG)
1.1	0.2	21.1	3.8	0
4.2	0.6	44.5	6.4	0
0.1	0.01	8.2	<1	0
5.9	0.9	39.4	6	0
0.02	0	<1	0	0
0	0	0	0	0
0.4	0.1	4.9	1.2	0
0	0	0	0	0
27	15	78.4	43.5	75
17.1	10.5	87.9	54	47
3.7	1.5	49.7	20.1	9
17.1	10.5	87.4	53.7	47
8.1	1.5	98.5	18.4	7
3.4	1.6	51	24	9
7.8	4.3	69.5	38.3	26
0	0	0	0	0
0	0	0	0	0
0	0	0	0	0
1.5	1	12.3	8.2	5
2	1	18	9	5
1.9	1.2	12.7	8	7
12	2	49.8	8.3	0

(continued)

FOOD	PORTION	CALORIES

ICE CREAM AND FROZEN TREATS (CONT.)

HIGH

FOOD	PORTION	CALORIES
Frozen yogurt, cherry, premium	½ cup	110
Ice cream, soft-serve, chocolate or vanilla, on cone	1 (about 5 oz)	230
Ice cream, vanilla		
reduced-fat	½ cup	130
regular	½ cup	170
Ice cream sundae, chocolate	1 (about 6 oz)	300
Ice milk, soft-serve, vanilla	½ cup	112

MEATS

BEEF

ACCEPTABLE

FOOD	PORTION	CALORIES
Steak, top round, lean, broiled	3 oz	153

HIGH

FOOD	PORTION	CALORIES
Brisket, lean, braised	3 oz	206
Corned beef hash, canned	1 cup	398
Ground, broiled		
extra-lean	3 oz	225
lean	3 oz	238
regular	3 oz	248
Liver, braised	3 oz	137
Meat loaf	3 oz	170
Roast		
bottom round, lean, braised	3 oz	178
pot, arm, lean, braised	3 oz	184
Shank cross cut, lean, simmered	3 oz	171
Short rib, lean, braised	3 oz	251

Fat (g)	Saturated Fat (g)	% Calories from Fat	% Calories from Saturated Fat	Cholesterol (mg)
2.5	**1.5**	20.5	**12.3**	10
7	**5**	27.4	**19.6**	20
4.5	**3**	31.2	**20.8**	35
10	**6**	52.9	**31.8**	105
7	**5**	21	**15**	20
2.3	**1.4**	18.5	**11.3**	7
4.2	**1.4**	24.7	**8.2**	71
10.9	**3.9**	47.6	**17**	79
24.9	**11.9**	56.3	**26.9**	73
13.4	**5.3**	53.6	**21.2**	84
15	**5.9**	56.7	**22.3**	86
16.5	**6.5**	59.9	**23.6**	86
4.2	**1.6**	27.6	**10.5**	331
11.2	**5.1**	59.3	**27**	55
7	**2.4**	35.4	**12.1**	82
7.1	**2.6**	34.7	**12.7**	86
5.4	**2**	28.4	**10.5**	66
15.4	**6.6**	55.2	**23.7**	79

(continued)

FOOD	PORTION	CALORIES

MEATS (CONT.)

BEEF (CONT.)

HIGH (CONT.)
Steak

filet mignon, lean, broiled	3 oz	179
flank, lean, broiled	3 oz	176
porterhouse, lean, broiled	3 oz	185
rib eye, lean, broiled	3 oz	191
sirloin, wedge bone, lean, broiled	3 oz	166
T-bone, lean, broiled	3 oz	182

LAMB

HIGH
Ground, broiled	3 oz	241
Kabob cubes, lean, broiled	3 oz	156
Leg, lean, roasted	3 oz	162
Rib roast, crown, lean, roasted	3 oz	197

LUNCHMEATS/PROCESSED MEATS

LOW
Turkey breast	2 slices (about 1½ oz total)	47

HIGH
Bologna		
beef	2 slices (about 2 oz total)	177
turkey	2 slices (about 2 oz total)	113
Chicken roll, light meat	2 slices (about 2 oz total)	90
Corned beef	2 slices (about 2 oz total)	142

FAT (G)	SATURATED FAT (G)	% CALORIES FROM FAT	% CALORIES FROM SATURATED FAT	CHOLESTEROL (MG)
8.5	3.2	42.7	16.1	71
8.6	3.7	44	18.9	57
9.2	3.7	44.8	18	68
10	4	47.1	18.8	68
6.1	2.4	33.1	13	76
8.8	3.5	43.5	17.3	68
16.7	6.9	62.4	25.8	82
6.2	2.2	35.8	12.7	77
6.6	2.4	36.7	13.3	76
11.3	4.1	51.6	18.7	75
0.7	0.2	13.4	3.8	17
16.2	6.9	82.4	35.1	33
8.6	2.9	68.5	23.1	56
4.2	1.2	42	12	28
8.5	3.5	53.9	22.2	49

(continued)

FOOD	PORTION	CALORIES

MEATS (CONT.)

LUNCHMEATS/PROCESSED MEATS (CONT.)

HIGH (CONT.)

FOOD	PORTION	CALORIES
Frankfurter		
beef	1	180
chicken	1	116
Ham, boiled, extra-lean	2 slices (about 2 oz total)	74
Liverwurst, fresh	3 slices (about 2 oz total)	185
Olive loaf	2 slices (about 2 oz total)	133
Pastrami		
beef	2 slices (about 2 oz total)	198
turkey	2 slices (about 2 oz total)	80
Pepperoni	10 slices (about 2 oz total)	273
Salami, pork	3 slices (about 2 oz total)	230
Sausage		
bratwurst, fresh	1 link (about 3 oz)	256
kielbasa, smoked	2 slices (about 2 oz total)	176
knockwurst, smoked	1 link (about 2½ oz)	209
pork, fresh	4 links (about 2 oz total)	192
scrapple	2 oz	120
Turkey ham	2 slices (about 2 oz total)	73

FAT (G)	SATURATED FAT (G)	% CALORIES FROM FAT	% CALORIES FROM SATURATED FAT	CHOLESTEROL (MG)
16.3	6.9	81.5	34.5	35
8.8	2.5	68.3	19.4	45
2.8	0.9	34.1	10.9	27
16.2	6	78.8	29.2	90
9.4	3.3	63.6	22.3	22
16.6	5.9	75.5	26.8	53
3.5	1	39.4	11.3	31
24.2	8.9	79.8	29.3	44
19.1	6.7	74.7	26.2	45
22	7.9	77.3	27.8	51
15.4	5.6	78.8	28.6	38
18.9	6.9	81.4	29.7	39
16.2	5.6	75.9	26.3	43
7.6	2.8	57	21	25
2.8	1	34.5	12.3	32

(continued)

FOOD	PORTION	CALORIES
MEATS (CONT.)		
PORK		
HIGH		
Bacon		
Canadian	2 medium slices (about 1½ oz total)	86
smoked	3 medium slices (about ¾ oz total)	109
smoked, thickly sliced	1 slice (about ⅓ oz)	50
Chop, center rib, lean, roasted	3 oz	208
Ham, cured, roasted	3 oz	140
Roast, center loin, lean, roasted	3 oz	204
Spareribs, lean, braised	3 oz	337
VEAL		
HIGH		
Ground, broiled	3 oz	146
Loin, lean, roasted	3 oz	149
MILK AND MILK PRODUCTS		
CREAM		
LOW		
Sour cream, fat-free	2 Tbsp	30
HIGH		
Half-and-half	2 Tbsp	39
Heavy	2 Tbsp	103
Light	2 Tbsp	59
Nondairy, powdered	1 tsp	10
flavored	1 tsp	60
Sour cream		
reduced-fat	2 Tbsp	35
regular	2 Tbsp	62

Fat (G)	Saturated Fat (G)	% Calories from Fat	% Calories from Saturated Fat	Cholesterol (MG)
3.9	1.3	40.8	13.6	27
9.4	3.3	77.6	27.2	16
4.5	2	81	36	10
11.7	4.1	50.6	17.7	67
6.5	2.2	41.8	14.1	48
11.1	3.8	49	16.8	77
25.8	10	68.9	26.7	103
6.4	2.6	39.5	16	88
5.9	2.2	35.6	13.3	90
0	0	0	0	2
3.5	2.2	80.8	50.8	11
11	6.9	96.1	60.3	41
5.8	3.6	88.5	54.9	20
0.5	0.5	45	45	0
3	2.5	45	37.5	0
2	1.5	51.4	38.6	10
6	3.8	87.1	55.2	13

(continued)

FOOD	PORTION	CALORIES
MILK AND MILK PRODUCTS (CONT.)		
CREAM (CONT.)		
HIGH (CONT.)		
Whipped cream	2 Tbsp	19
Whipped topping, nondairy	2 Tbsp	30
MILK		
LOW		
Dairy shake mix, chocolate, prepared with water	About 6 oz	80
Dry, nonfat, prepared	1 cup	82
Evaporated, fat-free	2 Tbsp	25
Fat-free	1 cup	86
ACCEPTABLE		
1% low-fat, chocolate	1 cup	158
HIGH		
Buttermilk	1 cup	99
Eggnog	½ cup	171
Evaporated	2 Tbsp	40
1%	1 cup	102
2%	1 cup	121
Whole	1 cup	157
Whole, chocolate	1 cup	208
YOGURT		
LOW		
Fruit		
light (low-calorie)	1 cup	100
regular	1 cup	240
Fruit with crunch-type topping		
light (low-calorie)	¾ cup	130
regular	¾ cup	220

Fat (g)	Saturated Fat (g)	% Calories from Fat	% Calories from Saturated Fat	Cholesterol (mg)
1.7	1	80.5	47.4	6
2.4	2	72	60	0
1	0	11.3	0	0
0.2	0.1	2.2	1.1	4
0	0	0	0	0
0.4	0.3	4.2	3.1	4
2.5	1.5	14.2	8.5	7
2.2	1.3	20	11.8	9
9.5	5.7	50	30	75
2	1	45	22.5	5
2.6	1.6	22.9	14.1	10
4.7	2.9	35	21.6	18
8.9	5.6	51	32.1	35
8.5	5.3	36.8	22.9	31
0	0	0	0	0
3	1.5	11.3	5.6	15
1	0	6.9	0	0
2	0.5	8.2	2	<5

(continued)

FOOD	PORTION	CALORIES
MILK AND MILK PRODUCTS (CONT.)		
YOGURT (CONT.)		
LOW (CONT.)		
Plain, fat-free	1 cup	120
HIGH		
Plain		
low-fat (1½% milk-fat)	1 cup	150
whole milk	1 cup	139
NUTS AND SEEDS		
NUTS		
LOW		
Chestnuts, European, roasted	1 oz	70
Filberts (hazelnuts), unblanched, dried	1 oz	179
ACCEPTABLE		
Almonds, unblanched, dried	1 oz	167
Pecans, dried	1 oz	189
Pistachios, dried	1 oz	164
Walnuts, English, dried	1 oz	182
HIGH		
Brazil, unblanched, dried	1 oz	186
Cashews, dry-roasted	1 oz	163
Coconut, sweetened, flaked	1 oz	126
Macadamia, dried	1 oz	199
Mixed, dry-roasted	1 oz	169
Peanuts, dry-roasted	1 oz	164
Pine, pignolia, dried	1 oz	146

Fat (g)	Saturated Fat (g)	% Calories from Fat	% Calories from Saturated Fat	Cholesterol (mg)
0	0	0	0	0
4	2.5	24	15	20
7.4	4.8	47.9	31.1	29
0.6	0.1	7.7	1.3	0
17.8	1.3	89.5	6.5	0
14.8	1.4	79.8	7.5	0
19.2	1.5	91.4	7.1	0
13.7	1.7	75.2	9.3	0
17.6	1.6	87	7.9	0
18.8	4.6	91	22.3	0
13.2	2.6	72.9	14.4	0
9	8	64.3	57.1	0
20.9	3.1	94.5	14	0
14.6	2	77.8	10.7	0
13.9	1.9	76.3	10.4	0
14.4	2.2	88.8	13.6	0

(continued)

Food	Portion	Calories

NUTS AND SEEDS (CONT.)

SEEDS

ACCEPTABLE

Food	Portion	Calories
Sunflower, dried	1 oz	162

HIGH

Food	Portion	Calories
Pumpkin, dried, hulled	1 oz	154
Sesame, dried, hulled	1 Tbsp	47

PASTA

LOW

Food	Portion	Calories
Fresh, cooked	1 cup	183
Macaroni, enriched, cooked	1 cup	197
Noodles		
egg, enriched, cooked	1 cup	213
soba, cooked	1 cup	113
spinach, enriched, cooked	1 cup	211
Spaghetti		
enriched, cooked	1 cup	197
whole wheat, cooked	1 cup	174
Spinach, fresh, cooked	1 cup	182
Vegetable, cooked	¾ cup	210

HIGH

Food	Portion	Calories
Tortellini, cheese	½ cup	220

DISHES

LOW

Food	Portion	Calories
Pasta salad with seafood, without dressing	3½ oz	90

ACCEPTABLE

Food	Portion	Calories
Lasagna with meat sauce, frozen	About 10 oz	270
Pasta primavera, frozen	About 10 oz	260
Spaghetti and meatballs, homemade	1 cup	332

FAT (G)	SATURATED FAT (G)	% CALORIES FROM FAT	% CALORIES FROM SATURATED FAT	CHOLESTEROL (MG)
14.1	1.5	78.3	8.3	0
13	2.5	76	14.6	0
4.4	0.6	84.3	11.5	0
1.5	0.2	7.4	1	46
0.9	0.1	4.1	<1	0
2.4	0.5	10.1	2.1	53
0.1	0.02	<1	<1	0
2.5	0.6	10.7	2.6	53
0.9	0.1	4.1	<1	0
0.8	0.1	4.1	<1	0
1.3	0.3	6.4	1.5	46
1	0	4.3	0	0
5	3	20.5	12.3	40
5	0.6	50	6	12
6	2.5	20	8.3	25
8	2.5	27.7	8.7	35
11.7	3.3	31.7	8.9	74

(continued)

Food	Portion	Calories

Pasta (cont.)

Dishes (cont.)

High

Fettuccine Alfredo, frozen	About 9 oz	270
Lasagna with meat sauce, frozen	About 10 oz	360
Macaroni and cheese, homemade, baked	1 cup	430
Manicotti, cheese, frozen	About 3 oz	290
Ravioli, cheese, with tomato sauce, frozen	About 9½ oz	360
Tortellini, cheese, with tomato sauce, frozen	About 9 oz	290

Pizza

Low

Cheese

Healthy Choice French bread pizza	1 (about 5½ oz)	310

Italian sausage

Healthy Choice sausage French bread pizza	1 (about 6 oz)	330
Supreme Lean Cuisine deluxe French bread pizza	1 (about 6 oz)	330

Acceptable

Cheese

Chef Boyardee, dry mix, prepared	1 slice (about 5 oz)	320
Weight Watchers extra cheese	1 (about 5¾ oz)	390

Pepperoni

Weight Watchers	1 (about 5½ oz)	390

Supreme

Weight Watchers deluxe combo	1 (about 6 ½ oz)	380

High

Cheese

Domino's thin crust	⅓ of 12″ pie (about 5½ oz)	364
Pizza Hut thin crust	1 slice of medium pie (about 3½ oz)	205

FAT (G)	SATURATED FAT (G)	% CALORIES FROM FAT	% CALORIES FROM SATURATED FAT	CHOLESTEROL (MG)
7	3	23.3	10	15
13	5	32.5	12.5	50
22.2	8.9	46.5	18.6	42
9	3.5	27.9	10.9	20
14	5	35	12.5	85
6	5	18.6	15.5	105
4	2	11.6	5.8	10
4	1.5	10.9	4.1	20
6	2.5	16.4	6.8	30
8	2.5	22.5	7	15
12	4	27.7	9.2	35
12	4	27.7	9.2	45
11	3.5	26.1	8.3	40
15.5	6.3	38.3	15.6	26
8	4	35.1	17.6	25

(continued)

FOOD	PORTION	CALORIES

PIZZA (CONT.)

HIGH (CONT.)

Italian sausage

Domino's hand-tossed, with mushrooms	2 slices of 12″ pie (about 6 oz total)	402
Pizza Hut hand-tossed	1 slice of medium pie (about 4 oz)	267

Pepperoni

Domino's hand-tossed	2 slices of 12″ pie (about 6 oz)	406
Healthy Choice pepperoni French bread pizza	1 (about 6 oz)	350
Pizza Hut hand-tossed	1 slice of medium pie (about 4 oz)	238

Supreme

Pizza Hut hand-tossed	1 slice of medium pie (about 5 oz)	284

Veggie

Domino's hand-tossed	2 slices of 12″ pie (about 6¾ oz total)	360
Pizza Hut hand-tossed	1 slice of medium pie (about 5 oz)	216

POULTRY, FOWL AND GAME

LOW

Chicken breast, without skin

fried in batter	½ (about 3 oz)	161
roasted	½ (about 3 oz)	142
Frogs' legs, uncooked	3 oz	62
Turkey		
breast, prebasted, roasted, without skin	3 oz	107
light meat, roasted, without skin	3 oz	34

Fat (G)	Saturated Fat (G)	% Calories from Fat	% Calories from Saturated Fat	Cholesterol (MG)
13.9	6.1	31.1	13.7	31
11	5	37	16	31
15.1	6.6	33.8	14.6	32
9	4	23.1	10.3	25
8	4	30.3	15.1	24
12	5	38	15.8	30
10.4	4.5	26	11.3	19
6	3	25	12.5	17
4.1	1.1	22.9	6.1	78
3.1	0.9	19.6	5.7	73
0.3	0	4.4	0	43
2.9	0.8	24.4	6.7	36
0.7	0.2	18.5	5.3	15

(continued)

Food	Portion	Calories

Poultry, Fowl and Game (cont.)

Acceptable

Food	Portion	Calories
Pheasant, meat only, uncooked	3 oz	113
Venison, roasted	3 oz	134

High

Food	Portion	Calories
Capon, roasted, without skin	3 oz	195
Chicken		
breast, with skin		
fried in batter	½ (about 5 oz)	364
roasted	½ (about 4 oz)	193
roasted, ready-to-serve	½ (about 5 oz)	250
drumstick, with skin		
fried in batter	1 (about 3 oz)	193
roasted	1 (about 2 oz)	112
liver, simmered	3 oz	133
thigh, without skin		
fried in batter	1 (about 2 oz)	113
roasted	1 (about 2 oz)	109
Duck, roasted, without skin	3 oz	171
Pâté		
chicken, canned	1 oz	57
goose, smoked, canned	1 oz	131
Potpie, turkey, homemade	1 piece (about 8 oz)	550
Rabbit, roasted	3 oz	131
Squab (pigeon), uncooked	1 (about 6 oz)	239
Turkey		
dark meat, roasted, without skin	3 oz	32
dark meat, roasted, with skin	3 oz	188
light meat, roasted, with skin	3 oz	168
liver, simmered	3 oz	144

Fat (g)	Saturated Fat (g)	% Calories from Fat	% Calories from Saturated Fat	Cholesterol (mg)
3.1	1.1	24.7	8.8	56
2.7	1.1	18.1	7.4	95
9.9	2.8	45.7	12.9	73
18.5	4.9	45.7	12.1	119
7.6	2.2	35.4	10.3	82
13	4	46.8	14.4	110
11.3	3	52.7	14	62
5.8	1.6	46.6	12.9	47
4.6	1.6	31.1	10.8	536
5.4	1.5	43	11.9	53
5.7	1.6	47.1	13.2	49
9.5	3.6	50	18.9	76
3.7	1.1	58.4	17.4	111
12.4	4.1	85.2	28.2	43
31.3	10.5	51.2	17.2	72
5.4	1.6	37.1	11	54
12.6	3.3	47.4	12.4	151
1.2	0.4	33.8	11.3	15
9.8	3	46.9	14.4	76
7.1	2	38	10.7	65
5.1	1.6	31.9	10	532

(continued)

Food	Portion	Calories

SOUPS AND STEWS

SOUPS

LOW

Food	Portion	Calories
Black bean, condensed, made with water	1 cup	116
Clam chowder		
Manhattan, condensed, made with water	1 cup	78
New England, low-fat	1 cup	120
Crab	1 cup	76
Gazpacho	1 cup	56
Minestrone, low-fat	1 cup	120
Onion, condensed, made with water	1 cup	58
Split pea with ham, low-fat	1 cup	170
Tomato		
condensed, made with water	½ cup	100
low-fat	½ cup	90
Vegetarian vegetable, condensed, made with water	1 cup	72

ACCEPTABLE

Food	Portion	Calories
Bouillon, chicken, from cube, made with water	1 cup	12
Chicken noodle, condensed, made with water	1 cup	75
Chicken rice, condensed, made with water	1 cup	60
Green pea, condensed, made with water	1 cup	165
Lentil with ham	1 cup	139

HIGH

Food	Portion	Calories
Beef noodle, condensed, made with water	1 cup	83
Beef vegetable, condensed, made with water	1 cup	78
Bouillon, beef, from cube, made with water	1 cup	7
Cheese, condensed, made with water	1 cup	156
Cream of celery, condensed, made with water	1 cup	90
Cream of chicken, condensed, made with water	1 cup	117
Cream of mushroom, condensed, made with water	1 cup	129

Fat (G)	Saturated Fat (G)	% Calories from Fat	% Calories from Saturated Fat	Cholesterol (MG)
1.5	0.4	11.6	3.1	0
2.2	0.4	25.4	4.6	2
2	0.5	15	3.8	5
1.5	0.4	17.8	4.7	10
2.2	0.3	35.4	4.8	0
2	0.5	15	3.8	<1
1.7	0.3	26.4	4.7	0
2.5	1	13.2	5.3	10
2	0	18	0	0
2	0.5	20	5	0
1.9	0.3	23.8	3.8	0
0.3	0.1	22.5	7.5	0
2.5	0.7	30	8.4	7
1.9	0.5	28.5	7.5	7
2.9	1.4	15.8	7.6	0
2.8	1.1	18.1	7.1	7
3.1	1.2	33.6	13	5
1.9	0.9	21.9	10.4	5
0.2	0.1	25.7	12.9	0
10.5	6.7	60.6	38.7	30
5.6	1.4	56	14	15
7.4	2.1	56.9	16.2	10
9	2.4	62.8	16.7	2

(continued)

FOOD	PORTION	CALORIES

SOUPS AND STEWS (CONT.)

SOUPS (CONT.)

HIGH (CONT.)

Cream of potato, condensed, made with water	1 cup	73
Scotch broth, condensed, made with water	1 cup	80
Turkey vegetable, condensed, made with water	1 cup	72

STEWS

HIGH

Beef, ready-to-serve	1 cup	194
Oyster, condensed, made with water	1 cup	58

VEGETABLES

LOW

Broccoli, boiled	½ cup	22
Cabbage, boiled, shredded	½ cup	17
Carrot, raw	1 (about 7½″, 2½ oz)	31
Chile peppers, raw, chopped	½ cup	30
Corn, sweet yellow, boiled	Kernels from 1 ear	83
Eggplant, boiled, cubed	½ cup	13
Garlic, raw	1 clove	4
Okra, boiled	½ cup	26
Onions, raw, chopped	½ cup	30
Pumpkin, canned	½ cup	41
Tomatoes, raw, chopped	1 cup	38
Zucchini, raw, sliced	½ cup	9

POTATOES

LOW

Baked		
plain, flesh only	1 (about 6 oz)	145
plain, microwaved, flesh and skin	1 (about 8 oz)	212

Fat (g)	Saturated Fat (g)	% Calories from Fat	% Calories from Saturated Fat	Cholesterol (mg)
2.4	1.2	29.6	14.8	5
2.6	1.1	29.3	12.4	5
3	0.9	37.5	11.3	2
7.6	2.5	35.3	11.6	34
3.8	2.5	59	38.8	14
0.3	0.04	12.3	1.6	0
0.3	0.04	15.9	2.1	0
0.1	0.02	2.9	<1	0
0.2	0.02	6	<1	0
1	0.2	10.8	2.2	0
0.1	0.02	6.9	1.4	0
0.02	0	4.5	0	0
0.1	0.04	3.5	1.4	0
0.1	0.02	3	<1	0
0.3	0.2	6.6	4.4	0
0.6	0.1	14.2	2.4	0
0.1	0.02	10	2	0
0.2	0.04	1.2	<1	0
0.2	0.1	<1	<1	0

(continued)

FOOD	PORTION	CALORIES
VEGETABLES (CONT.)		
POTATOES (CONT.)		
LOW (CONT.)		
Boiled, flesh only	1	67
Sweet potato, baked	1 (about 4 oz)	117
ACCEPTABLE		
Mashed, made with whole milk and margarine	½ cup	111
O'Brien	½ cup	79
Potato salad	½ cup	179
HIGH		
Au gratin	½ cup	161
Baked, with sour cream and chives	1 (about 6 oz)	221
French fries		
deep-fried	20–25 1″–2″ strips	235
frozen, oven-heated	20 (about 4 oz total)	222
microwave	1 box (about 3 oz)	230
Potato pancake	1 (about 3 oz)	234
Scalloped	½ cup	105

FAT (G)	SATURATED FAT (G)	% CALORIES FROM FAT	% CALORIES FROM SATURATED FAT	CHOLESTEROL (MG)
0.1	0.02	1.3	<1	0
0.1	0.03	<1	<1	0
4.4	1.1	35.7	8.9	2
1.2	0.8	13.7	9.1	4
10.3	1.8	51.8	9.1	85
9.2	5.8	51.4	32.4	28
12.6	5.6	51.3	22.8	14
12.2	3.8	46.7	14.6	0
8.8	4.5	35.7	18.2	0
12	3	47	11.7	0
12.6	3.4	48.5	13.1	93
4.5	2.8	38.6	24	15

WILLIAM P. CASTELLI, M.D., is medical director of the Framingham Cardiovascular Institute, a wellness program at Metro West Medical Center in Massachusetts. He is a former director of the Framingham Heart Study, which now encompasses five generations of Framingham townspeople, and coauthor of *Good Fat, Bad Fat: How to Lower Your Cholesterol and Reduce the Odds of a Heart Attack.*

INDEX

Underscored page references indicate boxed text and tables.